Contents

Acknowledgements

THE AUTHORS would like to thank the following people for their patience and invaluable help: Georgina West for typing the recipes; Sue Brenchley, Stella Bowling, Jane Bebell, Sue Bosanko and Judith North for their valuable comments; Elaine Messenger for putting a great deal of time and effort into evaluating the recipes; and Anise Kanji, Hanif Ladha and Joanne Winter for typing the text.

And thanks to our husbands, Shamil and Kieron, for being so tolerant!

RECIPES FOR HEALTH

Diabetes

Low fat, low sugar, carbohydrate counted recipes for the management of diabetes

AZMINA GOVINDJI AND JILL MYERS

Thorsons
An Imprint of HarperCollins*Publishers*

Thorsons
An Imprint of HarperCollins*Publishers*
77–85 Fulham Palace Road,
Hammersmith, London W6 8JB
1160 Battery Street,
San Francisco, California 94111–1213

First published as *The Essential Diabetic Cookbook*
by Thorsons 1992
This edition revised and updated 1995
9 10 8

© Azmina Govindji and Jill Myers 1992, 1995

Azmina Govindji and Jill Myers assert the moral right to
be identified as the authors of this work

A catalogue record for this book
is available from the British Library

ISBN 0 7225 3139 7

Typeset by
Harper Phototypesetters Limited, Northampton, England
Printed and bound in Great Britain by
Caledonian International Book Manufacturing Ltd, Glasgow

Foreword

FOOD IS ONE of life's great pleasures. Having diabetes does not and need not change that. People with diabetes should know that they can enjoy any food they want. They must bear in mind just two constraints – quantity and timing.

Diabetes is having too little insulin action and, therefore, too much sugar. Food and insulin are closely linked. When the person without diabetes eats a meal, the pancreas gland automatically delivers into the bloodstream just enough insulin to process the foodstuffs for the body. People with diabetes can no longer do this. They need an 'insulin assist'. Some may be able to boost their own diminished insulin supply with a tablet, while others produce so little that they have to inject it from a syringe.

For people injecting insulin, the dose and meal need to be in balance to control and prevent wide swings – upwards or downwards – of the amount of glucose in the blood. Often, the insulin is injected just before the meal so that the two meet together. With tablets the link is not quite so close, but meal timing is important to prevent the blood glucose falling to very low levels (hypoglycaemia). For overweight people, the dietitian will advise a reducing diet – all the foods but less of them.

All this must sound complicated, even menacing to the newly diagnosed diabetic – not exactly a prescription for carefree mealtime enjoyment. However, once the initial shock has passed, a few simple facts absorbed and confidence restored, normal food and interesting meals are emphatically back on the agenda. That's when *Recipes for Health: Diabetes* comes into play. It is full of delicious dishes, aromatic advice, mouthwatering morsels. At the same time, it is a painless guide to healthy and hearty eating for the whole family.

The two authors of the book, Azmina Govindji and Jill Myers, are both very experienced in their fields. Azmina Govindji, Chief Dietitian of the British Diabetic Association, has been actively involved in the development of guidelines for diet in diabetes since 1987. As Assistant Head of the Diet Information Service, she maintains close links with government bodies, academic institutions, health professionals, food manufacturers and the media. Azmina offers advice on all matters relating to food and diabetes.

Jill Myers, formerly Home Economist to the British Diabetic Association, has considerable experience in recipe development and cookery demonstrations. While at the Association she was responsible for the production of a range of tried and tested recipes for people with diabetes and for catering establishments. She was the primary source of advice on recipe modification. Jill Myers is now working for a major food retailer as a home economist developing quality own label foods.

Whether you cook it or just eat it, with the help of this book you can look forward to pleasurable culinary ventures and enjoyable mealtimes. So, read on and *bon appetit!*

Professor Harry Keen, MD, FRCP
Chairman, Executive Council,
British Diabetic Association,
Professor Emeritus, United Medical
and Dental School, Guy's Hospital Campus

1

What's So Special about This Book?

YOU MAY never need another cookbook. Why not? Because this book tells you all you need to know about food now that you have diabetes. It is not just another cookery publication. This book

- is the most up-to-date cookery book for people with diabetes, incorporating all the latest dietary policies from the British Diabetic Association
- contains a wide variety of high-fibre, low-fat, low-sugar recipes that are in line with the general principles of healthy eating. This means it provides attractive recipes and essential information not only for people with diabetes, but also for anyone wishing to lose weight or to eat more healthily
- has something for everyone – the elderly who need to prepare quick, easy, and possibly cheap meals; students living on limited budgets; parents who want to provide nutritious food for the family; the keen cook who invites guests with diabetes to dinner;

vegetarians and vegans; the weight watcher; and, of course, the person with diabetes

- is a comprehensive guide to diabetes and its dietary treatment.

Sections include information on choosing the right mix of foods, healthy eating for the whole family, watching your weight, eating out, what to do in an emergency and lots more. Then there are over 200 recipes to help you put it all into practice. From soups and starters to tasty meat, fish and vegetarian dishes, this book is a must for anyone who wants to cook everyday food in an appetizing way. And who said people with diabetes shouldn't eat. puddings? The mouthwatering pudding and dessert recipes will certainly prove that you need not compromise on taste just because you have diabetes!

Introducing Diabetes

WHAT IS DIABETES?

Diabetes mellitus (commonly known as diabetes) affects about two per cent of the UK population, and over 30 million people worldwide. In people with this condition, the amount of glucose in the blood is too high because the body is unable to use it properly. Glucose comes from the digestion of starchy foods such as bread or potatoes, from sugar and other sweet foods, and from the liver which makes it and passes it into the bloodstream. Insulin, a hormone produced by the pancreas, helps the glucose to enter the cells where it is used as fuel by the body.

The main symptoms of untreated diabetes are increased thirst, passing large amounts of urine, extreme tiredness, blurred vision, weight loss and itching of the genitals.

Insulin dependent diabetes (also known as Type 1 diabetes) occurs when there is a severe lack of insulin in the body because most or all of the cells which produce it have been destroyed. This type of diabetes usually appears before the age of 40. It is treated by insulin injections and diet.

Non-insulin dependent diabetes (also known as Type 2 diabetes) occurs when the body can still produce some insulin, though not enough for its needs, or when the insulin that the body does produce is not used properly by the body. This type of diabetes usually appears in people over the age of 40 and often in those who are overweight. It is treated by diet alone or by diet and tablets or, occasionally, by diet and insulin injections.

The two main aims of treatment are to eliminate the symptoms and to prevent long-term complications, such as eye, nerve, kidney and foot problems.

Diet is the foundation for the management of diabetes and the control of symptoms, and following a sensible food plan will help to keep your blood sugar close to the normal range. This in turn helps to reduce the risk of developing long-term complications. The diet for diabetes is not a special one in any way: it is a healthy eating pattern which is recommended for everyone, with or without diabetes, and one that the whole family can enjoy.

You will be able to adapt your usual meals to make them more healthy. Foods that you thought you would have to give up – such as cakes and desserts – do not need to be cut out completely. They can be eaten occasionally, as part of an overall healthy diet. Eating a variety of healthy foods can give you a sense of well-being and vitality.

The information in this book covers the basic guidelines for diabetes. For further information, contact your local Diabetic Association (see Useful Addresses, on page 284).

Don't worry if all you've heard about eating well is that carrots help you see better in the dark and spinach gives you iron – just read on.

If you have diabetes, remember to:

- continue with your treatment even if symptoms have disappeared
- attend the clinic for regular check-ups.

YOUR FEELINGS

Being told that you have a condition which will last for the rest of your life is bound to have an effect on how you organize the practical aspects of daily living and also on your feelings. It is natural for you, your family and your friends to feel sad about the loss of spontaneity that diabetes can sometimes cause. Perhaps you feel angry, asking yourself, 'Why me?' and maybe you are worried about the future.

At times like this, talking to other people who also live with diabetes can be a great help. They can share their experiences with you and give you support. The team at your diabetes clinic may be able to put you in contact with other people with diabetes. Also, your local Diabetic Association will know people who you can contact and may also arrange local support groups.

There are people with diabetes in all walks of life –

from professional sports people to politicians. Some of them will work in occupations or follow interests *you* want to pursue. Although you will have to think ahead a little more than you did before, don't feel that having diabetes prevents you from having a full life.

HEALTHY EATING

Why is it so important to eat healthily? Research studies worldwide suggest that watching what you eat is not only essential to the management of diabetes, but that it can also help prevent heart disease, constipation, bowel problems, obesity and tooth decay. Following a good diet also makes you feel good!

There is no such thing as a bad food; there is only a bad diet. All foods can have some nutritional benefit, but it is the mix of foods and the amounts you eat that make what you eat healthy or unhealthy.

In diabetes, the nutrient value of a food is not the only consideration. The way a particular food is digested and its effect on blood sugar can influence the general control of diabetes. For example, mashed potatoes can make blood sugar rise quicker than the same amount of boiled potatoes, simply because vegetables that are left whole take longer to digest.

The following general guidelines on healthy eating will also help you to choose the right types of food. You don't need to do everything at once; start by choosing those ideas you find the easiest and gradually try to bring in the others.

- Eat regular meals and try to eat similar amounts of starchy foods from day to day.
- Try to eat more high-fibre foods. The fibre in beans, peas, lentils, vegetables, fruit and oats is particularly good.
- Cut down on fried and fatty foods such as butter, margarine, fatty meat and cheese.
- Reduce your sugar intake by swapping high-sugar foods for low-sugar foods.
- Try to get to the weight that is right for you and stay there.
- Be careful not to use too much salt.

The following suggestions will help you to put all this into practice, while the recipes in this book will enable you to prepare your favourite foods in a healthier way.

1. *Eat regular meals and try to eat similar amounts of starchy foods from day to day.* If you take insulin or tablets for your diabetes, keeping fairly closely to regular mealtimes can help to avoid hypoglycaemia (low blood sugar). Even if you do not take medication, you will find that your diabetes is easier to control if you have three or so small, regular meals a day rather than one or two large meals.

Make starchy foods (such as bread, potatoes, cereals, rice and pasta) the main part of your meal and try to eat roughly the same amounts from day to day.

2. *Try to eat more high-fibre foods.* Fibre is the part of food you don't digest. Fibre-rich foods are important for the

prevention and treatment of constipation. And as they are filling and generally low in calories, they are useful if you are trying to lose weight. Fibre is found in foods such as wholemeal and wholegrain bread, jacket potatoes, wholegrain cereals, fruits and vegetables.

In diabetes, foods high in a particular type of fibre – soluble fibre – can improve blood glucose (sugar) control. Research has shown that the soluble fibre found in oats, beans and lentils can slow down the rise in blood glucose levels after a meal, so it makes sense for people with diabetes to eat these foods frequently. Soluble fibre can also reduce abnormally high blood cholesterol. Some of the recipes that follow, such as the Chick Pea Moussaka (see page 140), demonstrate how you can use such foods to cook a substantial and appetizing meal.

Current nutritional thinking recommends that everyone include more fibre in their diet.

When you increase your intake of fibre, do so gradually: a new style of eating should never be adopted in haste. Drink more fluids, too, in the form of water or low-calorie drinks because your body needs plenty of fluid to digest fibrous foods. Try to drink at least six to eight cups a day.

Ways of Eating More Fibre

- Choose wholemeal, wholegrain or granary bread, vegetables with a skin (such as jacket potatoes, sweetcorn, peas), beans, lentils, brown rice and high-fibre breakfast cereals (such as porridge, muesli, bran-based cereals) in preference to more refined low-fibre foods.
- Substitute fruit juice with fresh fruit (a glass of apple

juice has around 100 kcalories and no fibre whereas
an apple provides only about 40 kcalories and has 2
grams of fibre).

- Choose foods as close to their natural state as possible.
  A food that is refined or processed generally contains
  less fibre. For example, white flour is lower in fibre
  than wholemeal flour, which has been made from the
  whole of the wheat grain.
- Keep high-fibre foods as whole as possible, having
  boiled or baked potatoes rather than mashed, and
  make a whole bean casserole (such as the Mixed Bean
  Hot Pot on page 142) instead of a puréed lentil soup.
  Such foods are digested more slowly and this helps to
  keep blood sugar levels steady.
- Try to use more beans, peas and lentils. They are
  cheaper than meat and are a good source of protein
  and fibre. Tinned baked beans are a quick way of
  getting more fibre and you don't even need to buy the
  sugar-free variety – the ordinary ones contain an
  insignificant amount of sugar.

Take 5!

Nutrition experts all over the world are now promoting
the 'Take 5' message: take 5 portions of fruit and vegetables a day. This recommendation is based on studies
which have shown that a high intake of fruit and vegetables may be associated with lower rates of heart disease
and cancer. As well as soluble fibre, fruits and vegetables
contain protective antioxidant vitamins – vitamins C, E
and beta carotene.

Both the British Diabetic Association (BDA) and the World Health Organisation (WHO) recommend a daily intake of at least 400 grams (1 pound) of fruit and vegetables. This does not include potatoes and can be achieved by eating five portions of fruit and vegetables a day.

Choose fruit more often as an in-between meal snack and eat plenty of vegetables.

3. *Cut down on fried and fatty foods*.

A high fat intake has been shown to increase your chances of becoming obese (very overweight) or of developing heart disease. It therefore makes sense to cut down on the amount of fatty foods you eat regardless of whether or not you have diabetes. There are three main types of fat:

- saturated fats, such as dairy products, animal fats
- monounsaturated fats, such as olive oil, rapeseed oil, peanut oil
- polyunsaturated fats, such as corn oil, sunflower oil, fish oil.

Cholesterol

Cholesterol is a fatty substance that forms an essential part of the body's cells, but, equally, too much cholesterol in the body can cause problems. If the level of cholesterol in your blood is too high, you increase your chances of developing heart disease. Cholesterol can build up in the arteries (the large blood vessels) in the heart. This accumulation of cholesterol can eventually cause the arteries to become completely blocked, leading to a heart attack.

Some foods are high in cholesterol, but cutting down on these alone does not make a significant difference to blood cholesterol levels. It is more important that you cut down on the amount of *saturated* fat that you eat, as eating too much saturated fat increases your blood cholesterol level. This is particularly important for people with diabetes, as they are more prone to heart problems.

The unsaturated fats do not raise blood cholesterol in the same way that saturated fats do. Evidence now suggests that monounsaturated fats can also help keep blood cholesterol levels low. A lot of monounsaturated fat in the form of olive oil is eaten in the traditional diets of most Mediterranean countries and the rate of heart disease in these countries is low, so it would seem that the diet may be one of the factors responsible for this. Studies in other countries have also shown that healthy diets low in saturated fat and high in monounsaturated fat may reduce the risk of developing heart disease. There seems, therefore, to be an advantage in substituting foods that are high in saturated fat with polyunsaturated and monounsaturated alternatives, as well as reducing your total fat intake.

Remember that *all* fats and oils are high in calories, so use only small quantities and choose monounsaturated or polyunsaturated types whenever possible.

Fish Oils

Rates of heart disease are also low in countries where fish is eaten in large quantities. It is thought that this is because of a particular type of fat contained in fish oils. It has not yet been absolutely proved, but you certainly have nothing to lose by eating more fish. Oily fish such as mackerel, herring, salmon and trout are an excellent source of protein and of vitamins A, D and E. Try to replace some of your meat intake with fish (especially oily fish) to improve the overall quality of your diet while helping you to cut down on your total fat intake. How about making Smoked Mackerel Pâté (see page 59)?

Fats and Figures

Remember that fat is a very concentrated source of calories, so eating less fat can help you lose weight. (Calories are units used to measure the energy values of foods – see Counting Calories on page 17 for more information.) One boiled egg is approximately 70 kcalories. Have it fried and the calories almost double. A tablespoon of oil is approximately 100 kcalories – this is about the same number of calories as half a pint of beer. Think about this when you see an oily dressing on a salad!

Low-fat foods can play an important role in reducing the total amount of fat in your diet. Whether you are watching your weight, need to eat less for a specific medical condition or are simply trying to avoid a heart attack, low-fat foods can make life much easier. However, be careful not to rely too heavily on some of them (such as low-fat sausages, low-fat cream cheese, low-fat crisps) because they still provide a lot of calories. Furthermore, low-fat spreads are not fat-free, so don't use twice as much! All the recipes in this book encourage low-fat cooking methods.

How to Eat Less Fat

- Try to avoid frying foods – grill, bake, boil, poach or steam instead.
- Butter and all margarines contain about the same amount of fat. Choose a reduced or low-fat monounsaturated or polyunsaturated spread. Ordinary low-fat spreads are also a good substitute for butter.
- Use lower fat versions of dairy products, for example, semi-skimmed or skimmed milk, half-fat cheddar, cottage cheese, low-fat yogurt, fromage frais.
- Cut down on fat-containing snack foods such as crisps, cakes, chocolates and biscuits.
- Buy lean meat or trim the fat off fatty meat. Poultry can be low in fat if the skin is removed. Eat fish more often. Oily fish is high in polyunsaturated fat, but, remember not to fry it!
- Watch out for processed foods that are high in fat, such as pies and other meat products – read the label.
- If you need to use oil in cooking, use as little as possible. Choose one that is high in monounsaturated fat (such as olive oil, rapeseed oil, peanut oil) or polyunsaturated fat (such as corn oil, sunflower oil, safflower oil, soya oil). Experiment with using olive oil by trying the Courgette and Sweetcorn Gratin (see page 149) or Red Lentil Lasagne (see page 133) recipes.

4. Reduce your sugar intake by swapping high sugar foods for low sugar foods.

It is often thought that sugar is needed for energy. However, energy is also derived from starch, protein and fat – in fact, every type of food we eat provides us with energy. All we get from sugar is calories. Sugar contains no useful nutrients nor has it any special energy-giving properties over other foods. In people with diabetes, sugary foods can cause blood glucose to rise rapidly, which is undesirable. Sugary foods can also lead to tooth decay, particularly if they are eaten between meals. Also, as sugar-containing foods are often high in fat and low in fibre, eating too many chocolates, desserts and cakes can make you put on weight.

Much of the sugar we eat is added by food manufacturers. Some packaged foods may be high in sugar even when they appear to be healthy, such as cakes and biscuits bought from health food shops. The ingredients list may not even specify sugar – but watch out for words like maltose, dextrose, honey, treacle, golden syrup, fructose, and corn syrup on the label. All of these are types of sugar and are not significantly better for you than ordinary standard sugar. Remember, too, that sucrose is simply the chemical term for ordinary standard white table sugar.

Get into the habit of reading labels and choosing foods that are low in *all* forms of sugar. If an item is low down on the ingredients list, there is less of that ingredient in the food than the ingredients given before it.

Sugar can cause tooth decay and eating too many

sugary foods can make you put on weight, so eat less sugar.

Sugar and Diabetes – Putting it into Context

People with diabetes are advised to avoid drinks containing sugar. Because the sugar in these drinks is in liquid form, it can enter the blood quite quickly. This causes blood sugar to rise rapidly. With diabetes, you want to avoid this.

However, if sugar is taken mixed in with food (such as an ice-cream after a meal), then blood sugar rises more slowly. So, if you wish to eat a small amount of sweet food, such as a piece of cake or a dessert, then try to have it after a meal.

Cutting Down on Sugar

- Try not to add sugar to drinks or cereals. There is a range of artificial sweeteners that make excellent substitutes (see Artificial Sweeteners, page 16).
- Choose unsweetened fruit juice, and diet or low-calorie drinks rather than sweetened soft drinks. One 330ml can of a sweetened fizzy drink can contain 7 teaspoons of sugar!
- Buy reduced-sugar jams, pure fruit spreads and fruit tinned in natural juice instead of their sweetened alternatives.
- Save cakes, sweets and chocolates for special occasions only.
- Look at labels and try to avoid manufactured foods that contain a lot of sugar.

Artificial Sweeteners – not Sugar, but Sweet

Artificial sweeteners have made an enormous range of foods readily available for all those who want to avoid large quantities of sugar – slimmers, the health conscious and people with diabetes. They impart an intense level of sweetness and are virtually calorie-free. Available as tablets, liquids or in granulated form, they can be used to replace sugar in drinks, cereals and puddings. They are also found in many reduced-calorie foods such as diet yogurts, low-calorie squash and diet soft drinks.

All these artificial substitutes for sugar are food additives and so are required by law to undergo rigorous tests for safety before being approved for use. Examples of those commonly used are aspartame, saccharin, and acesulfame potassium (acesulfame K). All of these are widely available under various brand names. Neo-hesperidine (NHDC) is the newest permitted sweetener in this country. Cyclamate is widely sold in Europe and may receive approval for sale in the UK.

Personal preferences vary, so it is a good idea to shop around until you find one that suits your palate and your pocket best – the prices also vary! If you tend to use a lot of sweeteners in drinks, cereals, puddings and processed foods, make sure you vary the type of sweetener you choose so as to reduce any chance of over-consumption of one food additive.

Unlike sugar, artificial sweeteners do not cause tooth decay and are virtually calorie-free.

5. *Try to get to the weight that is right for you and stay there.*
If you are underweight, you may not be getting all the
nutrients you need. If you are overweight, your diabetes
will be harder to control.

Counting Calories

What Are Calories?
The term 'calories' or 'kcalories' (kilocalories) is used to
describe the amount of energy provided by the food you
eat. All food provides calories but some foods are more
concentrated in calories than others. For example, a
100g/4oz apple will provide you with around 50 kcalories, whereas a 100g/4oz piece of Cheddar cheese would
provide 400 kcalories. This is because every food
contains a different proportion of fat, carbohydrate and
protein. Weight for weight, fat contains twice as many
calories as either carbohydrate or protein. Therefore,
those foods that have a higher percentage of fat are likely
to be highest in calories.

On food labels, the calorific value of a food is usually
written as kcal/100g. For example, if a label states 350
kcals/100g then this means that a 100g/4oz portion of the
food would provide 350 kcalories. You may also see the
term kilojoule (kj) used on labels. One kcalorie is equal to
4.2kj.

If the number of calories you take in from the food you
eat is the *same* as the number you use up in your daily
activities, your weight should be more or less stable.
However, if you take in *more* calories from food than you
use up, you are likely to gain weight. On the other hand,

Introducing Diabetes

if you eat *less* than normal but maintain your usual level of activity, you may lose weight.

Why Count Calories?

Being overweight can increase your chances of developing diabetes, heart disease and high blood pressure. If you have diabetes and are overweight, weight reduction can improve the control of your diabetes and may even mean that you can reduce the dosage of your medication.

Motivation

Why is it that at some time in their lives most people have tried some sort of slimming diet, that the bookshops are oozing with novel ideas on how to shed those extra pounds and yet obesity is *still* a major problem in most Western countries?

From the restricted grapefruit diet (not to be encouraged) to the more sensible high-fibre, low-fat type of diet, you are presented with hundreds of ways to cut down on calories. Often one of these will help you lose weight but, more often than not, the weight starts to creep back on again. There are, no doubt, many reasons for this, but one of the most important is motivation – or lack of it. If you can maintain your motivation, then you are more likely to make a concerted effort to persevere. How, though, can you keep yourself motivated? It is unlikely that you will keep to a diet if it makes unreasonable demands on your normal lifestyle. Only if your new way of eating fits in with your social habits, your time constraints, your budget and your food preferences will you have a strong chance of keeping your weight down for a significant length of time.

Support

Reputable commercial slimming clubs can provide invaluable personal support as you try to lose weight. Most people who are trying to lose weight need guidance on more than just what to put on their plates at mealtimes. Psychological and emotional support can make changing your eating behaviour much easier and often these clubs can provide a degree of one-to-one counselling.

In some cases, your doctor may refer you to the state registered dietitian at the local hospital or clinic. A qualified dietitian will take your medical history, age, sex and lifestyle into account and will then be able to help you with a personal food plan. This can vary from person to person. The dietitian can, in addition, offer guidance and support as necessary.

If you follow the general guidelines on healthy eating given on pages 6–8 you will be able to adopt a style of eating that will help you lose weight while still providing you with all the nutrients you need. If you choose the foods you eat sensibly and cook them in the ways suggested in this book, you will be able to reduce your calorie intake and still enjoy tasty, filling meals.

Sensible slimming suggestions

• Be realistic when deciding how much weight you want to lose – setting a goal that seems unattainable could make you feel frustrated and give up.

- Set short-term targets and reward yourself once you've reached them. For example, treat yourself to a record or a book after you've lost 7 lb (about 3kg). Don't use food as a reward, though, or you'll undo all your good work!
- Try recording *exactly* what you eat – you may be surprised to see how the nibbles and snacks mount up.
- Make changes slowly. For example, try to avoid fried foods one week and, then, in the following week, to eat high-fibre breakfast cereals as well.
- Write down your successes – this can help keep you motivated.
- Try to encourage your family to eat healthily. This way you won't need to prepare foods specifically for yourself, you will simply need to have smaller portions.
- Think of ways to help your meals appear larger. Use a smaller plate, or have a selection of vegetables.
- Try to avoid TV dinners as concentrating on TV can make you less aware of how much you're eating. Try to sit down when you are eating – it's amazing how much you can munch your way through on the move!
- Don't shop when you're hungry – you may be tempted into buying more than you need (using a shopping list is a good idea) and avoid the aisles full of sweets and biscuits and the cakes at the in-store bakery!

Are You Overweight?

It's obviously worth finding out if you *need* to lose weight before you start slimming. Use the chart on page 22 to estimate how much (if any) weight you need to lose.

Remember not to make unreasonable demands on yourself. Aim to get down to a weight that is practical and possible. Don't bother to weigh yourself every day as you may find you lose one day and gain the next. This is normal, but can be disheartening. Try to weigh yourself only once a week and at around the same time of day.

Diets that offer a weight loss of 7 lb (3kg) in a week may sound like a miracle cure, but will not help you in the long term. So be patient – it took time to gain the excess weight, so losing it effectively is going to take time, too. The ideal rate of weight loss is around 1–2 lb (½–1kg) per week, although there is often a rapid loss in the beginning (mostly of water). A steady weight loss of around 4 lb (2kg) per month is good.

As time goes on your body adapts to your new calorie intake by needing fewer calories for normal functions such as breathing. Don't be discouraged, keep at it. Keep up the motivation, maintain variety, experiment with new recipes, reward yourself (but not with food) when you have done well, exercise, eat out (sensibly) on occasions, take up a new hobby, diet with a friend or whatever else helps. Do everything within your power to get down to that target weight – it will be worth it.

Weight Chart

Take a straight line across from your height (without shoes) and a line up from your weight (without clothes). Mark where the two lines meet.

From Garrow JS (1981), *Treat Obesity Seriously*. Edinburgh: Churchill Livingstone.

Underweight Maybe you need to eat a bit more, but go for well-balanced nutritious foods and don't just fill up on fatty and sugary foods. If you are *very* underweight, see your doctor about it.

OK You're eating the right *quantity* of food but you need to be sure that you're getting a healthy *balance* in your diet.

Overweight You should try to lose weight.

Fat You need to lose weight.

Very fat You urgently need to lose weight. You would do well to see your doctor, who might refer you to a dietitian.

If you need to lose weight, aim to lose 1 or 2 lb (½–1kg) a week until you get down to the 'OK' range. Go for fibre-rich foods and cut down on fat, sugar and alcohol. You'll need to take regular exercise too.

Use the recipes in this book to help you follow the healthy eating guidelines. Each recipe has been given a calorie value to help you keep track of how much you are eating.

If you have insulin dependent diabetes, changing your diet may mean you have to inject less insulin. It is best to consult your doctor and dietitian before adopting a reduced calorie, and probably carbohydrate, diet.

What happens next? Often after getting your weight down successfully, it slowly starts to creep up again as you allow yourself more treats. Once you are satisfied with your weight, gradually include more variety, especially of the high fibre starchy foods. Start, for example, by having an extra slice of bread or an extra helping of potatoes and then slowly introduce more of the other foods you enjoy. Continue to step on the scales regularly so that you can keep your new weight in check.

Lastly, good luck – you *can* do it!

6. *Be careful not to use too much salt.*
Most experts on nutrition advise you to eat less salt. Why?

In some people, eating salt may be linked with high blood pressure. Although a small amount of salt is needed by the body, it is possible for the average person to eat up to ten times more salt than the body requires. A lot of the salt we eat is added by the manufacturers during food processing. Cutting down on processed food can therefore help you to eat less salt.

Cutting Down on Salt

- Use less salt in cooking (experiment with other seasonings, such as herbs and spices).
- Avoid adding salt at the table.
- Eat fewer salty manufactured foods, such as smoked and preserved meat and fish, sausages and salted snack foods.

What about Alcohol?

Weight for weight, alcohol contains more calories than sugar, so even moderate drinking can make you gain weight. For example, one pint of beer has about the same number of calories as three chocolate biscuits. Also, as

These drinks all contain roughly the same amount of alcohol.

½ pint ordinary beer = *single measure of spirits = small glass of sherry = glass of wine = 1 unit

*In Northern Ireland a single measure of spirits = 1½ units.

alcohol contains negligible nutrients, it is of little dietary benefit. Replacing meals with alcoholic drinks can make you lose out on important vitamins and minerals. If you have diabetes, you don't need to give up drinking alcohol altogether, but you do need to think more carefully about what you drink and when.

Alcohol in large quantities can damage your liver. The recommended maximum intake for anyone, with or without diabetes, is 3 units of alcohol for men and 2 units for women. Try to have two or three drink-free days each week. Pregnant and breastfeeding women should ideally avoid alcoholic drinks altogether.

The above all contain one unit of alcohol.

Use the guidelines below to help you keep your social drinking to safe limits.

- Do not exceed the recommended maximum intakes.
- Try low-sugar, low-alcohol drinks – they are better for your blood glucose (important if you have diabetes) and for your waistline.
- Never drink on an empty stomach; eat before you drink.

Introducing Diabetes

- Alternate your alcoholic drinks with alcohol-free drinks. If drinking spirits, use sugar-free mixers or soda water.
- Remember not to drink and drive.
- If you have diabetes, you should also note the following:
  - you may drink up to three units of sweet wine or sherry as part of your weekly allowance, but try not to drink them all on the same occasion
  - you should avoid the special low-carbohydrate beers and lagers that were originally brewed for people with diabetes – they are higher in alcohol and calories than ordinary beers
  - it is important to wear some form of diabetic identification – you and others may confuse low blood sugar (hypoglycaemia) with drunkenness
  - alcohol lowers blood sugar, so remember this, particularly if you are on insulin. This (hypogly-caemic) effect can last several hours
  - if you count how much carbohydrate (CHO) you eat, don't include the CHO from alcoholic drinks.

About Carbohydrate

The amount of carbohydrate (CHO) or starchy foods eaten daily is an important consideration for people with diabetes. It is often felt that people with diabetes should cut down on starchy foods. This is not true. In the past, a low CHO diet was encouraged. However, it has since been shown that if around half your daily calorie intake comes from high-CHO, high-fibre foods, then your blood sugar level will improve. This is obviously better in the long term. The starchy foods recommended in the section on fibre on pages 7–9 are the best types to choose. The soluble fibre they contain has the most favourable effect on blood glucose and may also help reduce blood cholesterol levels.

Latest Developments
Many studies have been conducted in this field and you may hear rumours that this amount of CHO can make your control worse, instead of improving it. Don't worry! After an extensive review of all the research that has been published, the British Diabetic Association still recommends that a high-CHO, low-fat diet is the most appropriate for people with diabetes, *provided the diet is high in soluble fibre*, particularly in its whole, unprocessed form. The Canadian, Australian, American and European Associations also encourage a high-CHO, high-fibre, low-fat diet.

What is a 'CHO exchange'?
All meals eaten by people with diabetes must contain some CHO. To help people with diabetes control their CHO intake and still enjoy varied and interesting meals, a system of 'exchanges' has been developed. An exchange refers to a particular amount of CHO. One apple and one orange each contain approximately 10g of CHO, and can thus be 'exchanged', or swapped, for one another.

CHO 'exchange lists' are used by some insulin dependent diabetics, but they can be impractical. Many people prefer to use ordinary household measures (cups, spoons and so on) to weigh food. It may be that general advice on the quantity of the diet and the best mix of foods will eventually replace the CHO counting system. Placing so much emphasis on CHO is considered by many experts to be misleading as CHO is not the only nutrient that you need to adjust when you have diabetes. Far more important is the *whole diet*: the mix of foods that are eaten and when, how long they are cooked and whether they are puréed or eaten whole.

Exchange lists are, however, still very much in use. In Canada and America, in fact, up to nine food exchange lists may be used. The European Association for the Study of Diabetes, while currently recommending CHO exchange systems, acknowledges that better exchange lists should be developed. These lists should encourage the use of the more beneficial type of CHO, high-soluble fibre carbohydrates.

Each recipe in this book has been given a carefully calculated CHO value – this will be useful to you if your dietitian has prescribed a daily CHO allowance.

Use this book to ensure that you select the foods that are the most appropriate for good control of your diabetes and also for good health.

Diabetic Products

These specialist products have been on the market since the 1960s. At that time, the diabetic diet strictly prohibited the consumption of sugar and a low carbohydrate intake was encouraged. Because of this, special diabetic foods that were sugar-free and low in carbohydrate were considered to be a good idea.

Times change, however, and, as we learn more about nutrition, so do recommended diets. Today a high-carbohydrate, high-fibre diet is recommended and a small amount of sugar is acceptable, provided that it forms part of this diet. So treats can now include ordinary chocolates, cakes or biscuits, so long as they are eaten in small amounts within the context of a healthy diet, preferably at the end of a meal. Useful proprietary products that are not marketed especially for people with diabetes are sugar-free drinks, diet yogurts and artificial sweeteners.

So, you don't *need* to buy or eat special diabetic products. Because they also tend to be expensive and are often no lower in fat or calories than their non-diabetic equivalents, consuming them is now discouraged in many countries.

MAKING MEALS

You now know which foods are the better ones to choose and which foods to cut down on; you will shortly learn which cooking methods to adopt and have a selection of tasty recipes, but how do you transform all this knowledge and information into practical food terms? How do you 'make meals'?

Here is an example of a day's food intake. Have a go at changing the foods chosen and the cooking methods so that the meals are healthier and more appropriate for people with diabetes. Then turn the page to find a possible solution – see how your suggestions compare.

A day's food	Healthier choices

Breakfast
Cornflakes with whole
milk and sugar   _____
White toast with butter
and jam   _____
Coffee with milk and sugar   _____

Lunch
2 slices white bread with
Cheddar cheese, tomato
and mayonnaise   _____
Banana   _____
Sugary fizzy drink, such
as Coke   _____

Mid-afternoon snack
2 chocolate biscuits   _____
Tea with milk and sugar   _____

Supper
Shepherd's pie   _____
Cabbage   _____
Fruit crumble   _____
Custard   _____

Bedtime
Tea with milk and sugar   _____

Healthier choices	Comments
Breakfast	
Breakfast cereal containing bran or porridge or muesli	• more fibre • oats contain soluble fibre
Semi-skimmed or skimmed milk	• less fat
Granulated artificial sweetener	• sugar free
Wholemeal or granary toast	• whole grains may help keep blood sugar at a safe level
Polyunsaturated or monounsaturated	• less saturated fat
margarine or low-fat spread	• less total fat and fewer calories
Reduced-sugar jam or pure fruit spread	• less sugar • fewer calories
Coffee with semi-skimmed or skimmed milk	• less fat
Artificial sweetener	• sugar free
Lunch	
2 slices wholemeal or granary bread	• more fibre
Low-fat or half-fat cheddar or cottage cheese or Edam cheese	• less fat
Tomato	

Healthier choices	Comments
Reduced-calorie mayonnaise	• less fat and fewer calories
Banana	
Diet fizzy drink (such as diet Coke or equivalent)	• sugar free and fewer calories

Mid-afternoon snack

2 plain biscuits	• less sugar, less fat and fewer calories
Tea with semi-skimmed or skimmed milk	• less fat and fewer calories
Artificial sweetener	• sugar free

Supper

Lean savoury mince	• less fat
Boiled or baked potatoes in their jackets	• more fibre
	• vegetables kept whole
Sweetcorn	• more soluble fibre
Fruit crumble, sweetened with artificial sweetener and crumble topping made from wholemeal flour, muesli, poly- or mono-unsaturated margarine or low-fat spread	• sugar free
	• more fibre (muesli has soluble fibre)
	• less saturated fat or less total fat

Bedtime

| Tea with semi-skimmed or skimmed milk | • less fat |
| Artificial sweetener | • sugar free |

As you can see, only small changes have been made, but by choosing low-fat, high-fibre, low-sugar foods and by adopting sensible cooking methods, the health giving quality of the meals has been greatly improved. Use this guide and the practical cooking tips on pages 47–9 to help you make all your meals more healthy.

THE PLATE MODEL –
THE LATEST APPROACH

You eat foods, not nutrients. It is helpful to translate all this advice into what you actually put on your plate. For this reason, many health experts, including the British Diabetic Association, have issued guidelines on how much of your plate should be filled by individual foods. Such an approach provides a visual guide to meal planning.

Always make starchy foods such as bread, potatoes, rice, pasta or cereals the main part of your meal. More than a third of your plate should be covered by this filling starchy food (see plate diagram overleaf). Around the same amount of your plate should contain vegetables (and/or fruit). The remainder of your plate is left for the protein foods, such as meat, fish, cheese or eggs. This amounts to about a quarter of the area on your plate and will help you to cut down on fat and calories. Even if you are not concerned about your calorie intake, these proportions are considered to be ideal for general health.

Starchy foods

Fruit and vegetables

Protein foods

EATING AWAY FROM HOME

If you have diabetes, there is no reason why you can't visit the local fast food joint, the posh restaurant in town, go to your friend's house for dinner or a holiday resort abroad.

A Quick Take-Away

As with any food or drink, it makes sense to limit the amount of 'fast food' you eat. It does have the benefit of being quick and convenient, so avoiding it altogether can be a nuisance. Simply try not to rely on such foods too often and, when you do, make the most healthy choice possible. For example, choose a smaller hamburger in a wholemeal bun, if available, and unsweetened orange juice or a diet drink. Try to resist that sugary, processed apple pie. They are often more like apple fritters than pies and can be incredibly high in fat. Remember, too, that one milkshake can have more calories than seven wine glasses of fresh orange juice!

The Chinese stir-fry is becoming an increasingly popular fast-food choice. These foods are generally healthy, particularly since a wide variety of vegetables make up an important part of the meal. Obviously the oily dishes such as deep fried seaweed, spring rolls, fried prawn balls, crispy Peking duck and fried noodles can be very high in fat, and steamed alternatives are preferable. The main meals generally contain very little carbohydrate and only the rice and noodle dishes need to be counted if you are on a daily carbohydrate allowance. Sweet and sour dishes are best kept for special occasions. They tend to be high in fat, sugar and calories.

The Greek doner kebab may look lean, but have you noticed the oil that trickles down the outside? Don't believe you have lost all of the fat in this way, there is still 'hidden' fat in the meat. Lower fat choices are grilled kebabs, especially chicken. Fill some hot pitta bread (preferably wholemeal) with kebabs and a colourful salad for a filling, nutritious and convenient meal.

The local 'chippy' unfortunately does not have many healthy foods on offer since most items are deep fried or contain pastry. Ordering a couple of rolls and less of the fatty food can be helpful.

The tempting aroma emanating from an Indian restaurant can act like a magnet when you are hungry! Choose lentil (or dahl) based dishes, tandooris and grills, naan or chapati (unbuttered) and boiled rice. Save high fat dishes like fried poppadums, butter chicken, paratha (deep fried Indian bread) and biryani or pilau rice for special occasions. Did you know that an average portion of pilau rice has more than double the calories of a portion of plain boiled rice?

Dining in Style

What about a night out at an exclusive restaurant? On a special occasion, why not enjoy yourself and eat what you like? If it is your birthday, anniversary, Christmas, whatever, do you think it will do you much harm to forget the fat and fibre for just one evening? If you want a small serving of dessert, remember that sugar has a less drastic effect on your blood sugar level when it is mixed in with lots of other ingredients and eaten at the end of a meal. (Remember if you take insulin, though, that you may need to make some adjustments – see page 37).

If you eat out frequently, however, perhaps attending business lunches or spending three nights a week wining and dining, then you need to think more carefully about the foods you choose. Try to avoid rich, creamy sauces, fried foods and sweet, fattening desserts. Watch the amount of alcohol you have, too.

Guess Who's Coming to Dinner?

When a friend invites you to dinner, don't forget that other people's knowledge of diabetes and food may be limited. If you feel that you would like to plan ahead, it may be worth letting your host or hostess know which foods you would prefer to be served – perhaps some of the mouthwatering dishes from this book! Otherwise, simply select whatever you think best from the dining table and, remember, an occasional lapse from your diet is not detrimental.

Sun, Sand, Sea – and Food

A little thoughtful planning before setting off for a week in the sun can make an important difference to your trip. Many people nowadays prefer self-catering accommodation, which will obviously mean that you have maximum control over what you eat. However, hotels often have a reasonable choice on the menu. If you are confronted with a range of unusual foods you are not sure about, you can almost always ask for bread, pasta or rice with a simple accompaniment like an omelette or cheese until you have discovered exactly what is on offer.

Remember to take extra carbohydrate supplies with you on the journey to your holiday destination. Suitable convenience snacks include sandwiches, fruit, biscuits and crisps. Take emergency supplies of glucose tablets or sweets along as well.

Insulin and Carbohydrate when eating out

If you take insulin, adjustments may need to be made to:

- your preceding snack or meal
- your insulin dose
- the timing of your injection.

You will probably work out what sort of changes are required by trial and error, but the following tips may be useful:

- plan ahead whenever possible
- extra carbohydrate (CHO) does need extra insulin (the dose depends on how much CHO is in the food)
- extra insulin is usually taken in the form of a quick-acting insulin shortly before a meal– this is particularly helpful if the meal is served later than you had anticipated
- you could delay the timing of your insulin injection if your meal is due to be taken later than usual
- if you are eating late, you could try having a snack at your usual mealtime to prevent your blood sugar from falling too low before your main meal
- if you use a pen injector, you will have a greater degree of flexibility – you can assess the CHO value of your meal and inject accordingly
- if you are dining and dancing, remember that the energy you use up while dancing will lower your blood sugar and, consequently, you may need to inject less insulin or eat more carbohydrate
- alcohol lowers blood sugar. Normally this is not a problem, but if you take insulin, it is important to have some food before or with an alcoholic drink and, most importantly, afterwards (such as a bedtime snack). This will prevent your blood sugar level falling too low, as the effect of alcohol can last for several hours.

EMERGENCY MEASURES FOR
LOW BLOOD SUGAR

The medical term for a low blood sugar level is hypoglycaemia or a hypo. Hypos are most likely to occur in
people who inject insulin, but some people on certain
tablets may also experience a hypo. It can be caused by:

- missing a meal or snack
- eating less carbohydrate than usual
- engaging in strenuous activity that you have not
  compensated for by, for example, eating some
  carbohydrate
- injecting more insulin than you need
- drinking alcohol on an empty stomach.

Please don't feel that you have to look for a cause,
however, as there may be no obvious reason.

Signs and symptoms of hypoglycaemia vary from one
person to the next, but common ones include light-
headedness, a faint feeling, sweating, shaking, hunger
and confusion. You will soon learn the warning signs
of a hypo and it is a good idea to let a friend or rela-
tive know what these are, too, so that they can recognize
one.

What to Do if You Have a Hypo

The main aim is to raise your blood sugar level quickly.
The fastest way to do this is to have some form of concentrated sugar (see the list on page 41 for examples)

immediately, followed by a snack, such as a slice of bread, biscuits or milk.

Carry something from the list below with you at all times. Wearing some sort of diabetic identification is an effective way of telling people you don't know around you that you have diabetes, should you need further help in such instances. If you cannot swallow, a doctor or ambulance should be called immediately. If you know why the hypo occurred, try to make adjustments to prevent it happening again. Seek the advice of your doctor, diabetes specialist nurse or dietitian if necessary.

ILLNESS

When you are ill, you may not feel like eating. However, even if you do not eat any food, you will find that your blood sugar level tends to go up when you are ill. Your body naturally responds to illness by making more sugar. It is obviously very important, therefore, to *continue with your diabetic treatment*. The following suggestions may also be useful:

- consult your doctor, particularly if you are vomiting
- if you are not eating, take fluids such as fruit juice, soup or a glucose drink (such as Lucozade), with 'a little and often', being a good motto – for example, half a glass every hour
- if you are eating, have small, frequent meals
- if possible, test your blood sugar or urine at least four times a day and keep a record of the results

- if you take insulin, the dose may need adjusting – for example, if your blood sugar is very high, you will need more insulin (call your doctor if you need help with this)

Suggested emergency items	Amount to take
Glucose tablets	3 tablets
Sugar or glucose powder	2 teaspoons
Sugar cubes	2 cubes
Honey, jam or syrup	2 teaspoons
Lucozade or similar glucose drink	50ml/2fl oz
Sugared fizzy drink, such as ordinary coca-cola	½ glass
Orange juice	½ glass

3

About the Recipes

ALL THE RECIPES in this book have been prepared in a healthy way. High-fibre, low-fat ingredients have been used and low-fat cooking methods have been chosen. Each recipe has been carefully tried and tested. The calorie and carbohydrate content of each recipe has been accurately calculated using the latest professional nutrition data.

THE INGREDIENTS USED

Fat
- wherever possible, polyunsaturated and monounsaturated oils (try to use monounsaturated oils more often)
- low-fat spread (including polyunsaturated low-fat spread)
- lean meat and poultry or low-fat dairy products.

Fibre
- lentils, beans, wholemeal pasta, brown rice, wholemeal flour, oats, dried fruit, fresh fruit and vegetables.

Sugar
- small amounts of ordinary sugar in baking
- artificial sweeteners in desserts where sugar is not required.

WEIGHTS AND MEASURES

Quantities of ingredients have been given in both metric and imperial measurements. The metric measurements have been used for the calculations. Choose whichever system of measurement you prefer, but use either *all* metric or *all* imperial, otherwise you risk a poor result, especially with pastry, breads and cakes.

RECIPE CALCULATIONS

All calculations are based on raw ingredients, unless the word 'cooked' appears in the ingredient list.

Carbohydrate (CHO) Calculations

The section about carbohydrate on page 26 explained why CHO is important in diabetes. Not all foods contain CHO. For example, many vegetables – such as lettuce, tomato, carrots and cabbage – and fruits – such as rhubarb, lemons, raspberries and gooseberries – have such small amounts of CHO that it does not make sense to count them (these are listed in Table 1, page 46). The same is true for flavourings such as stock and tomato purée. If a food contains less than 5g of CHO, it is considered negligible (referred to as 'neg.' in the recipes). The list below is of the vegetables that have been counted when making CHO calculations for the recipes in this book:

- baked beans
- pulses and beans, such as chick peas, split peas, lentils
- potatoes.

It is more practical to round up or down to the nearest 10g rather than to use the exact CHO value. For example if a recipe has 23g of CHO per portion, this has been rounded down to 20g. This makes CHO counting much easier.

Calorie calculations

All foods provide calories, but in some cases the number of calories is so minute that it is not necessary to count them. In this book, seasonings, certain condiments (such as vinegar and lemon juice) and artificial sweeteners have not been calorie counted.

Although some vegetables (such as cabbage and carrots) are very low in calories, their calorie content has been included in the recipe calculations to make them as accurate as possible. However, on a day-to-day basis the calories from these vegetables need not be counted, so eat them freely – choose from the list in Table 1 on page 46.

As with CHO, the exact calorie content of the ingredients has been assessed. The total figure for the recipe has then been rounded up or down to the nearest 10 kcalories.

ADAPTING YOUR OWN RECIPES
FOR HOME BAKING

No one is suggesting that you should throw away all your favourite recipes and cookbooks just because you are now following a healthy eating plan. Instead, modify them by reducing the amount of saturated fat and sugar they contain and increasing the amount of fibre. You may find the following guidelines useful:

- if a recipe calls for white flour, try using wholemeal flour instead or half wholemeal and half white. This gives a lighter texture than wholemeal on its own for sponge cakes and so on
- replacing butter and ordinary margarine with low-fat spread can reduce the fat and calories by half, but some of these spreads do not work well in baking, so polyunsaturated or monounsaturated margarines are a useful alternative. (Remember, however, that these margarines have exactly the same quantity of fat and calories as ordinary butter, although they do have the advantage of being high in unsaturated fat so using a polyunsaturated or monounsaturated low-fat spread gives you the best of both worlds; look out, too, for new low-fat products designed especially for baking)

- in most cases, you can reduce the sugar content of a traditional recipe (such as for a Victoria sandwich) by half: proportions of up to 50g/2oz of sugar to 225g/8oz of flour give satisfactory results in rock cakes, scones, fruit loaves and so on and, on average, this yields between 2 and 5g of sugar per scones, which is the same as a couple of digestive biscuits
- remember that if you use sugar, it does add to the carbohydrate content of a recipe
- not everyone needs to count their calories and CHO and you are certainly not expected to own food composition tables such as those that have been used in the compiling of this book, but if you are on a CHO allowance, the table below may be of help.

Ingredients	CHO (in grams)
25g/1oz flour (any kind)	20
25g/1oz sugar (any kind)	30
Polyunsaturated margarine or low-fat spread	No carbohydrate content
Eggs	No carbohydrate content
185ml/⅓ pint of milk (any kind)	10
25g/1oz dried fruit (any kind)	20
Up to 100g/4oz nuts	Negligible carbohydrate content
Up to 50g/2oz cocoa powder	Negligible carbohydrate content

PRACTICAL COOKING TIPS

- Try baking cakes using less sugar than a traditional recipe demands. In some cases you can use only half the normal amount and still concoct a mouthwatering treat. How about a Victoria Sandwich (see page 226) for a high-fibre, low-sugar accompaniment to afternoon tea?
- If making custard, use skimmed milk, custard powder and an artificial sweetener.
- Make your own jelly using low-calorie squash, unsweetened fruit juice and gelatine.
- Include beans, peas and lentils in recipes that contain meat. Replacing some of the meat with beans is cheaper and very nutritious.
- Use reduced or low-fat spread, preferably monounsaturated (if available) or polyunsaturated, for baking – try the Banana and Walnut Slices on page 230). Use non-stick cookware, too.
- Remove the skin from poultry and trim the fat off meat.
- Choose refreshing fruity desserts such as the Raspberry and Kiwi Whip on page 206, rather than rich stodgy puds.
- Reduce the amount of salt you use in cooking as we eat far more salt than we need. Flavour your food with lemon juice, herbs, spices or mustard instead for healthier, tastier food.
- Eat more oily fish, such as herring and mackerel, that are high in polyunsaturated fat and are still moist after grilling.

About the Recipes

- Grill, bake, poach, steam or boil foods rather than frying them. 25g/1oz of boiled potato provides about 20 kcalories – make this amount of potato into chips and the calories multiply three times!
- Choose oils that are high in monounsaturated fat (such as olive oil) or polyunsaturated fat (such as corn oil) and, even so, remember to use as little as possible. Also, remember that polyunsaturated oil becomes more saturated when it is reused, which makes it less desirable in your diet, but that monounsaturated oils are not altered when they are reused. So, when frying, choose a monounsaturated oil if you are planning to reuse it.
- Use low-fat dairy products in recipes, such as skimmed or semi-skimmed milk, reduced-fat cheese and low-fat yogurt. Low-fat cream cheese and low-fat yogurt make good substitutes for cream. How about making the Yogurt Gooseberry Fool on page 207?
- Beans don't necessarily need to be the dried variety, which require soaking. Canned beans are just as healthy and can be used straight away.
- Keep the skins on potatoes. This doesn't mean having potatoes baked in their jackets day in, day out – roasted, scalloped, sautéd or boiled potatoes can all be cooked with their skins on and you benefit from the extra fibre.
- Brown rice contains more fibre than white. Try it sometime. (Remember, though, that you need more water for brown rice and it takes longer to cook.)
- Use half wholemeal and half white flour for baking –

you don't need to use wholemeal on its own, which can be quite dry in some baked goods. Simply choose what you and your family find tastes good.

4

Soups and Starters

A N ENTICING starter often paves the way for good things to come. Starters should complement the main course. It's best to serve small portions and to present them attractively with eye-catching garnishes.

Cold starters can be prepared in advance, enabling you to deal with other parts of the meal or to take part in the socializing! Serve pâtés or dips with raw, fresh vegetables such as carrots, celery and cauliflower florets to help add fibre and colour.

Delicious, home-made soups are always welcoming on a cold winter's day. They are extremely nourishing and can be transformed into a light main meal if served with wholegrain granary rolls or bread. The use of vegetables and pulses in the soups helps to increase the fibre and adds texture.

TARAMASALATA

CHO 80g/kcalories 940
Serves 8–10

Metric/Imperial		American
8 small slices	wholemeal bread	8 small slices
175g/6oz	fresh smoked cod roe, skinned	1 cup
	juice of 1–2 lemons	
1 slice	onion	1 slice
1	clove garlic, crushed	1
50ml/2fl oz	oil	¼ cup
	olives, to garnish	

1. Soak the bread in water for 10 minutes. Squeeze it gently then put it in a food processor or blender.
2. Add the roe, lemon juice, onion and garlic. Blend for 2 minutes until well mixed.
3. Slowly add the oil while the blender is running. Blend for 1–2 minutes.
4. Serve with brown pitta bread and vegetable crudités.

Notes to Cooks

If a milder taste is preferred, add a little more bread and oil. If it is too stiff, add 1–2 teaspoons water. The consistently should be neither runny nor too stiff, but rather, a spreadable consistency.

Vegetable crudités is the French name for a dish of raw vegetables, including carrots, celery, cauliflower, peppers, radishes etc., usually cut into sticks and served with one or more dips or sauces as an appetizer or cock-tail snack.

MINESTRONE SOUP

CHO 50g/kcalories 790
Serves 6–8

Metric/Imperial		*American*
1 x 15ml sp/ 1 tbs	olive oil	
75g/3oz	rindless streaky bacon, chopped	3 slices
1	onion, chopped	1
1	clove garlic, crushed	1
3	stalks celery, chopped	3
2 small	carrots, finely chopped	2 small
1	courgette, chopped	1
25g/1oz	small dried pasta shells, bows or similar	¼ cup
	salt and freshly ground black pepper	
1 x 5ml sp/1 tsp	dried oregano or basil	1 tsp
1 x 15ml sp/ 1 tbs	tomato purée	1 tbs
1.1l/2 pints	chicken stock	5 cups
225g/1 x 8oz	can red kidney beans, drained and refreshed under cold running water	1¼ cups
	a little grated Parmesan cheese	

1. Heat the oil in a large saucepan. Add the bacon, onion and garlic and fry until the bacon is crisp.

2. Stir in the remaining vegetables (except the kidney beans) and pasta. Add seasonings, tomato purée and stock. Bring to boil, stirring constantly. Reduce the heat, cover and simmer for 20–25 minutes, stirring occasionally.
3. Add the kidney beans and simmer for a further 10 minutes or until all the vegetables are tender.
4. Adjust the seasoning to taste before serving and sprinkle with the Parmesan cheese.
5. Serve with bread or rolls.

TOMATO SOUP

CHO 20g/kcalories 380
Serves 4

Metric/Imperial		*American*
1 x 15ml sp/ 1 tbs	corn or sunflower oil	1 tbs
1 medium-sized	onion, peeled and chopped	1 medium-sized
2 rashers	streaky bacon, rinds removed and chopped	2 slices
1 x 15ml sp/ 1 tbs	flour	1 tbs
450g/1 lb	fresh tomatoes, halved and deseeded	1 lb
550ml/1 pint	chicken stock	2½ cups
	salt and freshly ground black pepper	
	pinch dried basil	
	lemon juice to taste	
1 x 5ml sp/1 tsp	intense sweetener	1 tsp

1. Heat the oil in a pan, add the onion and bacon and cook for 5 minutes.
2. Stir in the flour and cook for 1 minute, stirring constantly. Add the tomatoes and gradually stir in the stock.
3. Bring to the boil, then reduce the heat and add the seasonings. Simmer for 20 minutes.
4. Remove the pan from the heat and rub the soup through a sieve. Adjust the seasoning to taste, add lemon juice and sweetener then serve with bread or rolls.

LENTIL SOUP

CHO 50g/kcalories 430
Serves 4

Metric/Imperial		American
2	onions, peeled and chopped	2
3	carrots, chopped	3
100g/4oz	lentils	½ cup
1.1l/2 pints	ham stock	5 cups
	freshly ground black pepper	
	fresh parsley, to garnish	

1. Put the onions, carrots, lentils and stock in a pan.
2. Bring to the boil, then cover and simmer for 40–45 minutes, stirring occasionally.
3. Either liquidize the soup or rub it through a sieve. Adjust the seasoning to taste, then serve, garnished with parsley, with bread or rolls.

WATERCRESS AND ONION SOUP

CHO neg/kcalories 90
Serves 4

Metric/Imperial		*American*
1 bunch	watercress, washed and roughly chopped	1 bunch
2	onions, peeled and chopped	2
550ml/1 pint	vegetable stock	2½ cups
	a little grated nutmeg	
	salt and freshly ground black pepper	
	a few watercress leaves to garnish	

1. Put the watercress and onions in a pan. Add the stock and seasonings. Bring to the boil, cover and simmer for 20 minutes.
2. Leave to cool slightly, then pour the soup into a blender or liquidizer and blend until smooth.
3. Return the soup to the pan and reheat. Adjust the seasoning to taste.
4. Serve, garnished with the watercress, with bread or rolls.

TURKEY OR CHICKEN BROTH

CHO neg/kcalories 200
Serves 4

Metric/Imperial		*American*
1	chicken or turkey carcass and any leftover meat, diced	1
3	carrots, peeled and diced	3
2	leeks, thinly sliced	2
2 x 15ml sp/ 2 tbs	rice	2 tbs
1	bay leaf salt and freshly ground black pepper	1

1. Put the carcass in a large pan and cover with water. Add the remaining ingredients and bring to the boil.
2. Reduce the heat and simmer for 2 hours, skimming any froth and fat with a spoon when necessary. Add more water if the liquid in the pan becomes low.
3. Remove the carcass from the pan. Skim the soup well to remove any remaining fat and adjust the seasoning to taste, then serve with bread or rolls.

SMOKED MACKEREL PÂTÉ

CHO neg/kcalories 800
Serves 4

Metric/Imperial		American
225g/8oz	smoked mackerel fillets	½ lb
100g/4oz	skimmed milk soft cheese	½ cup
	or low-fat soft cheese	
	lemon juice to taste	
	salt and freshly ground	
	black pepper	

1. Flake the fish into a bowl. Add the soft cheese and lemon juice and season to taste. Mix the ingredients together well by hand or process in a liquidizer or blender.
2. Put the pâté into a serving dish and chill until needed.
3. Serve with melba toast.

Notes to Cooks

Will keep in refrigerator for up to 48 hours.

Melba toast is light and crisp and can be served instead of rolls with soup and other appetizers. It is made by cutting bread into thin slices and toasting slowly in the oven until crisp and golden. Alternatively, it can be made from thicker slices, toasted on both sides then split through the middle.

CHICKEN LIVER PÂTÉ

CHO neg/kcalories 430
Serves 4

Metric/Imperial		American
25g/1oz	low-fat spread	2 tbs
1 medium	onion, finely chopped	1
225g/8oz	chicken livers	½ lb
1 x 5ml sp/1 tsp	grated nutmeg	1 tsp
	salt and freshly ground black pepper	
1	slice lemon	

1. Put the low-fat spread in a pan and lightly sauté the onion for 1 minute. Add the chicken livers and seasonings. Continue cooking for 5–6 minutes, stirring occasionally. Leave to cool, then liquidize or blend until smooth.
2. Put the pâté into the serving dish and smooth the top. Put the lemon slice on top. Chill until needed.
3. Serve with melba toast.

Note to Cooks

Will keep in the refrigerator for up to 48 hours.

STUFFED PEARS

CHO 60g/kcalories 400
Serves 4

Metric/Imperial		American
2	dessert pears, cut in half, core removed and sprinkled with lemon juice	2
100g/4oz	cottage cheese	½ cup
25g/1oz	walnuts, chopped	3 tbs
1 x 15ml sp/ 1 tbs	raisins	1 tbs
few drops	Worcestershire sauce salt and freshly ground black pepper lettuce and tomato or lemon slices to garnish	few drops

1. Put the pear halves on a lettuce leaf. Put to one side.
2. Meanwhile, put the remaining ingredients in a bowl and mix them together well.
3. Pile the mixture into the pear halves and garnish with the tomato or lemon slices, then serve immediately.

GUACAMOLE

CHO neg/kcalories 510
Serves 4–6

Metric/Imperial		American
2	ripe avocados, about 100g/4oz/¼ lb each	2
1	lemon, juice of	1
1 small	onion, peeled and finely chopped	1 small
1	clove garlic, crushed	1
225g/½ lb	tomatoes, skinned, de-seeded and finely chopped	½ lb
dash of	Tabasco sauce freshly parsley, chopped to garnish	dash of

1. Scoop the flesh out from the avocados into a bowl. Mash the lemon juice into the flesh. Add the remaining ingredients and blend well until the mixture is quite smooth.
2. Chill until needed, then transfer it to a serving dish and sprinkle the parsley over it.
3. Serve with a selection of vegetable crudités or tortilla chips.

MEDITERRANEAN-STYLE MACKEREL

CHO neg/kcalories 820
Serves 4

Metric/Imperial		American
1 x 15ml sp/ 1 tbs	olive oil	1 tbs
1	onion, chopped	1
1	clove garlic, crushed	1
1 medium	aubergine, cut into small cubes	1 medium
2	tomatoes, chopped	2
1 x 5ml sp/1 tsp	oregano	1 tsp
1	mackerel, filleted salt and freshly ground black pepper	1

1. Heat the oil in a pan and sauté the onions and garlic until tender. Add the aubergine and cook for 5 minutes.
2. Add the tomatoes, seasonings and fish and simmer for 20 minutes.
3. Lift out the fish and put it on a serving dish. Serve it topped with the vegetables.

5

Meat and Poultry

FAMILY MEALS are often quite a challenge – making food that satisfies everybody's likes and dislikes and doesn't break the budget. We've put together a selection of some family favourites and adapted them so that they are healthier without sacrificing taste.

Inventive use of nourishing economical foods like the cheaper cuts of meat and fish, fresh vegetables in season and dairy products all help to produce delicious inexpensive meals.

Casseroles and stews are tasty, easy to make and to reheat if your family needs to have staggered mealtimes.

Another good idea is to add beans and other pulses to meat dishes. Not only does this increase the fibre but it makes the meat go further.

STUFFED PEPPERS AND TOMATOES

CHO 80g/kcalories 1570
Serves 4

Metric/Imperial		*American*
4	green peppers	4
4 large	tomatoes	4 large
2 x 15ml sp/ 2 tbs	tomato purée diluted in 150ml/¼ pint hot water	2 tbs
1 x 15ml sp/ 1 tbs	corn or sunflower oil	1 tbs

Stuffing

225g/8oz	lean, minced beef or lamb	½ lb
1 large	onion, chopped	1 large
150ml/¼ pint	hot water	3 cups
2 x 15ml sp/ 2 tbs	fresh parsley, finely chopped	2 tbs
	salt and freshly ground black pepper	
50g/2oz	brown rice, cooked	⅓ cup
50g/2oz	pine kernels	⅓ cup
50g/2oz	sultanas	⅓ cup

1. Cut a slice off the top of each pepper and tomato and reserve them. Deseed the peppers. Scoop out most of the tomato flesh, chop it and reserve it for the stuffing.
2. To make the stuffing, cook the meat and onions in a pan until they brown. Add the hot water, the reserved tomato flesh and seasoning ingredients. Mix well and

Meat and Poultry

65

cook for 15 minutes. Add the remaining ingredients, mix well and cook for 3 minutes. Arrange the tomatoes and peppers upright in a baking dish. Fill them with the stuffing, leaving a little room for it to expand and replace the reserved tops.

3. Pour the tomato purée mixture over them and cook at 375°F/190°C/gas mark 5 for 1 hour and 10 minutes, basting them occasionally. If all the liquid evaporates, add a few tablespoons of water.

BROCCOLI IN HAM AND CHEESE SAUCE

CHO 30g/kcalories 540
Serves 2

Metric/Imperial		American
225g/8oz	broccoli, cut into even-sized pieces	½ lb
25g/1oz	low-fat spread	2 tbs
25g/1oz	wholemeal flour	¼ cup
275ml/½ pint	skimmed milk	3¾ cups
50g/2oz	reduced-fat cheddar cheese, grated	½ cup
50g/2oz	lean ham, finely chopped	4 tbs
1 x 5ml sp/1 tsp	wholegrain mustard salt and freshly ground black pepper	1 tsp

1. Cook the broccoli until just tender but still crisp. Meanwhile, make the sauce.
2. Melt the low-fat spread over a low heat, add the flour and stir over the heat for 1 minute. Gradually add the milk, stirring, and bring to the boil. Reduce the heat and simmer for about 3 minutes. Reserve a tablespoon of the cheese and stir the remainder into the sauce. Stir in the ham, mustard and seasoning.
3. Arrange the broccoli in an ovenproof dish, pour the cheese sauce over it and sprinkle the reserved cheese over the top. Grill until the grated cheese melts and turns golden brown. Serve immediately with potatoes or bread.

PORK STIR-FRY

CHO neg/kcalories 790
Serves 4

Metric/Imperial		*American*
1 x 15ml sp/ 1 tbs	olive or sunflower oil	1 tbs
350g/12oz	lean pork tenderloin fillet, cut into thin strips	¾ lb
2.5cm/1 inch piece	root ginger, peeled and finely chopped	1 inch piece
1	carrot, peeled and diced	1
1	onion, peeled and finely chopped	1
2 small	courgettes, washed and sliced	2 small
100g/4oz	baby sweetcorn	⅔ cup
225g/8oz	beansprouts	4 cups
2 x 15ml sp/ 2 tbs	dry sherry	2 tbs
2 x 15ml sp/ 2 tbs	light soy sauce	2 tbs
	freshly ground black pepper	

1. Heat the oil in a wok or large frying pan. Add the pork, ginger and onion and stir-fry for 5 to 10 minutes or until the pork is cooked.
2. Add the carrot, onion, courgettes and corn and stir-fry for 5 to 10 minutes. Stir in the beansprouts, sherry and soy sauce. Mix well and stir-fry for 1 minute.
3. Season to taste with freshly ground black pepper and serve immediately with steamed rice or noodles.

Diabetes

SWEET-AND-SOUR CHICKEN

CHO 30g/kcalories 760
Serves 4

Metric/Imperial		*American*
1 x 15ml sp/ 1 tbs	olive or sunflower oil	1 tbs
3	boneless chicken breasts, skin removed, diced	3
1	onion, sliced	1
1	green pepper, deseeded and chopped	1
1	red pepper, deseeded and chopped	1
225g/1 x 8oz	can tomatoes	1 cup
225g/1 x 8oz	can pineapple pieces in natural juice	1½ cups
1 x 15ml sp/ 1 tbs	vinegar	1 tbs
1 x 15ml sp/ 1 tbs	soy sauce	1 tbs
	about 150ml/¼ pint/⅔ cup water	
	salt and freshly ground black pepper	

1. Heat the oil and lightly fry the chicken and onion for 5 minutes. Add the remaining ingredients.
2. Bring to the boil, stirring, cover and simmer for 20–30

minutes or until the chicken is tender, adding a little more water if it starts to get a bit dry.

3. Serve with rice and vegetable stir-fry.

STIR-FRIED CHICKEN WITH CASHEWS

CHO 30g/kcalories 1090
Serves 4

Metric/Imperial		American
4	boneless, skinless chicken breasts, cut into even-sized pieces	4
2.5cm/1 inch piece	root ginger, peeled and chopped	1 inch piece
2–3	cloves garlic, crushed	2–3
1–2 x 5ml sp/ 1–2 tsp	cornflour	1–2 tsp
1 x 15ml sp/ 1 tbs	dry sherry	1 tbs
1 x 15ml sp/ 1 tbs	light soy sauce	1 tbs
150ml/¼ pint	chicken stock	⅔ cup
1 x 15ml sp/ 1 tbs	olive or sunflower oil	1 tbs
50g/2oz	unsalted cashew nuts salt and freshly ground black pepper	3½ tbs

1. Put the chicken, ginger and garlic in a bowl and leave to stand. Meanwhile, mix the cornflour with the sherry, soy sauce and chicken stock.
2. Heat the oil in a large frying pan or wok. Add the nuts and stir-fry until they are lightly browned. Remove

them, then add the chicken, ginger and garlic and stir-fry until the chicken is cooked and tender.

3. Add the sherry, soy sauce and stock mixture and stir until the liquid has thickened. If the sauce becomes too thick, add a little water.

4. Season to taste with salt and freshly ground black pepper. Add the cashew nuts, mix them in well, heat it through, then serve immediately with vegetables and rice or noodles.

LEMON AND HERB BAKED CHICKEN

CHO neg/kcalories 370
Serves 2

Metric/Imperial		American
2	skinless, boned chicken breasts	2
½	lemon, juice of	½
2 x 5ml sp/2 tsp	olive or sunflower oil	2 tsp
1	clove garlic, crushed	1
	freshly ground black pepper	
pinch	mixed herbs	pinch

1. Score the chicken breasts with a sharp knife and lay them in an ovenproof dish.
2. In a small bowl, mix the lemon juice, oil, garlic, pepper and herbs.
3. Spoon the mixture over the chicken, leave to marinate for 30 minutes. Then bake at 375°F/190°C/gas mark 5 for 30 minutes, until the chicken is cooked.
4. Serve with new potatoes and vegetables.

CHICKEN BREASTS
WITH PINEAPPLE SAUCE

CHO 40g/kcalories 900
Serves 4

Metric/Imperial		*American*
1 x 220g/8oz	can pineapple slices in natural juice	1½ cups
1 x 15ml sp/ 1 tbs	olive or sunflower oil	1 tbs
4	boneless, skinless chicken breasts	4
1	onion, sliced	1
1	garlic clove, crushed	1
½	green pepper, deseeded and cut into strips	½
½	red pepper, deseeded and cut into strips	½
1–2 x 15ml sp/ 1–2 tbs	wine vinegar	1–2 tbs
3 x 15ml sp/ 3 tbs	tomato purée	3 tbs
275ml/½ pint	chicken stock salt and freshly ground black pepper	3¾ cups

1. Drain and cube the pineapple, reserving 4 table-spoons of juice.
2. Heat the oil over a moderate heat in a large saucepan, add the chicken and seal on all sides. Remove with a

slotted spoon, drain on kitchen paper and set aside.

3. Stir-fry the onion, garlic and pepper in the remaining oil for 2 minutes. Remove the vegetables with a slotted spoon and set aside.

4. Boil the vinegar in the pan until reduced to half the quantity. Stir in tomato purée and stock, return to the boil. Add the reserved pineapple juice, chicken and vegetables.

5. Season to taste, cover and simmer for 35 minutes or until chicken is cooked. If necessary adjust the seasoning, stir in the pineapple chunks, cover and cook for a further 10 minutes.

6. Serve with broccoli florets and vegetable rice (see page 197).

GREEK-STYLE LAMB KEBABS

CHO neg/kcalories 1820
Serves 4–6

Metric/Imperial		*American*
2 x 15ml sp/ 2 tbs	corn or sunflower oil	2 tbs
½	lemon, juice of	½
1–2	cloves of garlic, crushed	1–2
675g/1½ lb	boned leg of lamb, cut into cubes	1½ lb
	salt	
	cayenne pepper	

1. Beat the oil, lemon juice and garlic together and let the meat marinate in it for 4 hours, covered in a refrigerator, basting the meat occasionally.

2. Thread the meat onto skewers and grill for 8–10 minutes, turning the skewers to brown the meat on all sides. Brush the kebabs with the marinade once or twice. Allow an extra 5 minutes if cooking on a barbecue.

3. Season with salt and cayenne pepper to taste and serve immediately with salad and rice or pitta bread.

MINCED BEEF COBBLER

CHO 80g/kcalories 1140
Serves 4

Metric/Imperial		*American*
450g/1 lb	extra lean minced beef	1 lb
1	onion, peeled and chopped	1
2	carrots, peeled and diced	2
227g/1 x 8oz	cantomatoes	1 cup
about 150ml/¼ pint	beef stock	⅔ cup
	salt and freshly ground black pepper	

Cobbler

100g/4oz	fine self-raising wholemeal flour	1 cup
1 x 5ml sp/1 tsp	baking powder	1 tsp
	pinch salt	
25g/1oz	low-fat spread	2 tbs
150ml/¼ pint	skimmed milk	⅔ cup

1. Sauté the mince, onion and carrots in a saucepan until the mince is all lightly browned. Add the tomatoes and stock and simmer for 30 minutes, stirring occasionally. Season to taste with salt and freshly ground black pepper.
2. Meanwhile, rub the fat into the flour, baking powder and salt until the mixture resembles fine breadcrumbs, then stir in enough milk to form a soft dough.

Roll it out on a lightly floured surface until it is 1cm (½ inch) thick and, using a 5cm (2 inch) cutter, cut out circles.

3. Pour the mince mixture into an ovenproof dish and place the dough 'cobbles' around the edge, overlapping them. Brush them with the remaining milk and bake at 400°F/200°C/gas mark 6 for 10–12 minutes, until the cobbler has risen and turned golden brown. Serve immediately with peas and mashed potatoes, giving everyone a serving of the cobbler with their savoury mince.

BEEFBURGER SURPRISE

CHO neg/kcalories 700
Serves 4

Metric/Imperial		*American*
450g/1 lb	extra lean minced beef	1 lb
1	onion, peeled and finely chopped	
	salt and freshly ground black pepper	
50g/2oz	reduced-fat cheddar cheese, grated	½ cup

1. Put the mince, onion and seasonings into a bowl and mix them together well. Divide the mixture in half and shape each into an 18cm (7 inch) round. Sprinkle the cheese evenly over one round to within 1cm (½ inch) of the edges. Cover the cheese layer with the second round and pinch the edges together firmly, sealing the filling inside.

2. Cook the burger under the grill for approximately 6–8 minutes each side, or until cooked through. Cut it into quarters and serve in a brown roll with salad.

COTTAGE PIE

CHO 100g/kcalories 1190
Serves 4–6

Metric/Imperial		*American*
450g/1 lb	extra lean minced beef	1 lb
1	onion, peeled and chopped	1
2	carrots, peeled and finely chopped	2
227g/1 x 8oz	can tomatoes	1 cup
1 x 15ml sp/ 1 tbs	tomato purée	1 tbs
about 150ml/¼ pint	beef stock	⅔ cup
	salt and freshly ground black pepper	
600g/22oz	potatoes, peeled, boiled and mashed	2¾ cups

1. Sauté the minced beef, onions and carrots until the meat is all just brown, stirring occasionally. Stir in the tomatoes, tomato purée and stock. Season to taste with salt and freshly ground black pepper, cover and simmer for 30 minutes.
2. Spoon the mixture into an ovenproof dish and spread the mashed potato over the meat. Decorate the surface of the potato by drawing wavy lines on it with a fork.
3. Bake the pie in the oven at 375°F/190°C/gas mark 5 for 30–35 minutes. If liked, place the pie under the

grill just before serving to crispen the potato topping.

4. Serve with vegetables.

MACARONI MINCE

CHO 50g/kcalories 1130
Serves 4

Metric/Imperial		American
450g/1 lb	extra lean minced beef	1 lb
2 medium	onions, finely chopped	2 medium
1	clove garlic, crushed	1
1 medium	carrot, finely diced	1 medium
227g/1 x 8oz	can tomatoes	1 cup
	salt and freshly ground black pepper	
pinch	mixed herbs	pinch
about 150ml/¼ pint	beef stock	⅔ cup
225g/8oz	macaroni, cooked	4 cups
50g/2oz	half-fat hard cheese, grated	½ cup

1. Put the mince, onion, garlic and carrot in a pan and fry gently until all the mince has browned, stirring occasionally. Stir in the remaining ingredients and seasonings except the macaroni and cheese, bring to the boil and simmer for 20 minutes.
2. Once cooked, pour the macaroni into an ovenproof dish, put the mince over the macaroni and top with the grated cheese. Melt the cheese under the grill, then serve hot with vegetables or salad.

SPAGHETTI BOLOGNESE

CHO neg/kcalories 560
Serves 4

Metric/Imperial		American
350g/12oz	extra lean minced beef	¾ cup
1	onion, finely chopped	1
1	clove garlic, crushed	1
2	carrots, finely chopped	2
2	sticks celery, thinly sliced	2
100g/4oz	mushrooms, sliced	1½ cups
400g/1 x 14oz	can tomatoes, chopped, with juice	1¾ cups
1 x 15ml sp/ 1 tbs	tomato purée	1 tbs
150ml/¼ pint	beef stock	⅔ cup
1 x 2.5ml sp/ ½ tsp	basil	½ tsp
1 x 2.5ml sp/ ½ tsp	oregano	½ tsp
	salt and freshly ground black pepper	

1. Brown the minced beef in a large pan without added fat for 5 minutes. Drain off any excess fat, then add the onion, garlic, carrot, celery and mushrooms and stir well. Add the remaining ingredients and season to taste with salt and freshly ground black pepper. Bring to boil and simmer gently for 30–40 minutes, stirring occasionally.

2. While the Bolognese sauce is cooking, bring a large pan of salted water to the boil and cook the spaghetti. When the spaghetti is *al dente* and the Bolognese sauce is ready, drain the spaghetti and either add it to the sauce and mix well together or serve a nest of spaghetti on each plate, topped with the Bolognese sauce.

Note to Cooks

Remember to take into account the CHO values of any spaghetti. 45g cooked weight of wholemeal spaghetti = 10g CHO.

MOUSSAKA

CHO 140g/kcalories 1600
Serves 4–6

Metric/Imperial		American
1 large	aubergine (about 275g/ 10oz), sliced and sprinkled with 1 tsp salt	1 large
1 x 15ml sp/ 1 tbs	corn or sunflower oil	1 tbs
450g/1 lb	extra lean minced lamb	1 lb
1 large	onion, chopped	1 large
1	clove garlic, crushed	1
1 x 5ml sp/1 tsp	cinnamon	1 tsp
2 x 15ml sp/ 2 tbs	fresh parsley, chopped	2 tbs
	salt and freshly ground black pepper	
3 x 15ml sp/ 3 tbs	tomato purée	3 tbs
600g/22oz	potatoes, parboiled and sliced	3 cups

White sauce

25g/1oz	low-fat spread	2 tbs
25g/1oz	flour	¼ cup
275ml/½ pint	skimmed milk	3¾ cups
	salt and freshly ground black pepper	
pinch	ground nutmeg	pinch
1	egg yolk	1

1. Once the aubergines have rendered their bitter juices, pat them dry with absorbent kitchen paper. Heat the oil in a large frying pan and fry the aubergine slices until they are golden brown on both sides. Drain them on absorbent kitchen paper.
2. Meanwhile, sauté the lamb, onion and garlic until all the meat is brown. Add the cinnamon, parsley, salt and pepper to taste, tomato purée and a little water to moisten.
3. In a large, ovenproof casserole, put alternate layers of potatoes, meat and aubergines starting and ending with a potato layer.
4. Make the white sauce and allow it to cool slightly before mixing in the egg yolk. Spoon the sauce over the potatoes in the dish and bake at 375°F/190°C/gas mark 5 for 25–30 minutes or until the top is golden brown.

NAVARIN OF LAMB

CHO 10g/kcalories 1150
Serves 4

Metric/Imperial		American
1 x 15ml sp/ 1 tbs	corn or sunflower oil	1 tbs
1 large	onion, chopped	1 large
1	clove garlic, crushed	1
4	chump chops, trimmed of fat	4
1 x 15ml sp/ 1 tbs	flour	1 tbs
2	carrots, sliced	2
1 small	swede (about 225g/½ lb), peeled and chopped	1 small
1 x 15ml sp/ 1 tbs	tomato purée	1 tbs
400g/1 x 14oz	can chopped tomatoes	1¾ cup
1	bouquet garni	1
	freshly ground black pepper	
	fresh parsley, chopped, to garnish	

1. Heat the oil in a flameproof casserole. Add the onion and garlic and fry for 5 minutes.
2. Meanwhile, coat the lamb chops in the flour. Add them to the casserole and brown them quickly on both sides. Add the carrots, swede, tomato purée and tomatoes and bring to the boil.

3. Add the seasonings. Cover with a lid and transfer to oven and cook at 325°F/170°C/gas mark 3 for 1–2 hours, until the meat is tender. Adjust the seasoning to taste and sprinkle the chopped parsley over before serving with new potatoes or rice, plus vegetables.

BEEF STEW AND DUMPLINGS

CHO 100g/kcalories 2430
Serves 4

Metric/Imperial		*American*
2 x 15ml sp/ 2 tbs	corn or sunflower oil	2 tbs
675g/1½ lb	braising steak, trimmed and cut into cubes	1½ lb
3	sticks celery, sliced	3
3 small	carrots, peeled and sliced	3 small
1 small	swede (about 100g/4oz), peeled and cubed	1 small
2	onions, peeled and chopped	2
2 x 15ml sp/ 2 tbs	flour	2 tbs
2 x 15ml sp/ 2 tbs	tomato purée	2 tbs
500ml/1 pint	beef stock	2½ cups
2	bay leaves	
	freshly ground black pepper	

Dumpling mixture

100g/4oz	self-raising wholemeal flour	1 cup
50g/2oz	vegetable suet	⅓ cup
pinch	salt	pinch
1 x 15ml sp/ 1 tbs	parsley, chopped	1 tbs
	sufficient water to bind	

1. Heat the oil in a large, flameproof casserole. Add the meat and fry until it has browned to seal in the flavour (about 5 minutes). Add all the prepared vegetables and fry for 3 minutes. Stir in the flour and cook for 1 minute, stirring. Stir in the tomato purée, stock, bay leaves and seasoning and bring to the boil. Cover with the lid and bake at 350°F/180°C/gas mark 4 for 1–2 hours, until the meat is tender.

2. To make the dumplings, sift the flour into a bowl and stir in the suet, seasoning and parsley. Mix to a firm (not sticky) dough with water (about 5 tbs). Form into 8 dumplings and put them on top of the meat in the casserole for the last 20 minutes or so until the dumplings are light and fluffy (do not remove the lid during this 20 minutes).

CARBONADE OF BEEF

CHO 10g/kcalories 1640
Serves 4

Metric/Imperial		American
2 x 15ml sp/ 2 tbs	corn or sunflower oil	2 tbs
675g/1½ lb	chuck steak, cut into cubes	1½ lb
1	onion, peeled and chopped	1
4	celery stalks, chopped	4
2	carrots, sliced	2
1 x 15ml sp/ 1 tbs	flour	1 tbs
	salt and freshly ground black pepper	
1 x 5ml sp/1 tsp	vinegar	1 tsp
1	bouquet garni	1
275ml/½ pint	stout	1⅛ cups
	fresh parsley, chopped, to garnish	

1. Heat the oil in a flameproof casserole, then add the cubes of meat and brown them quickly on all sides. Add the vegetables and cook for 5 minutes. Stir in flour, seasonings, vinegar, bouquet garni and stout.

2. Cover the casserole and bake at 325°F/170°C/gas mark 3 for 1–2 hours, or until the meat is tender. Stir a little water into the casserole if it becomes dry during the cooking time.

3. Discard the bouquet garni and adjust the seasoning to taste just before serving with potatoes or bread.

Meat and Poultry

BARBECUED PORK CHOPS

CHO neg/kcalories 430
Serves 2

Metric/Imperial		American
2	lean pork chops or pork steaks	2

Barbecue sauce

1 x 15ml sp/ 1 tbs	chilli sauce	1 tbs
1 x 15ml sp/ 1 tbs	Worcestershire sauce	1 tbs
1 x 15ml sp/ 1 tbs	vinegar	1 tbs
1 x 15ml sp/ 1 tbs	tomato ketchup	1 tbs
1 x 5ml sp/1 tsp	light soy sauce	1 tsp
1	clove garlic, crushed	1

1. Mix the barbecue sauce ingredients together.
2. Put the chops or steaks in a casserole dish and bake at 375°F/190°C/gas mark 5 for approximately 10–15 minutes or until the chops are browned. Pour off any fat. Pour the sauce over them and re-cover. Bake for 25–30 more minutes, basting them occasionally.
3. Arrange them on a serving dish and spoon the sauce over them.
4. Serve with jacket potato and salad or rice and vegetables.

6

Fish

THERE ARE TWO main types of fish: the oily ones –
such as mackerel – and white fish – such as cod,
haddock and so on. The oils in oily fish are excellent
sources of vitamins A and D and are also thought to
protect the body against heart disease.

With the recipes in this chapter for both white and oily
fish, you can cook up a tempting feast that will also
benefit your general well-being.

TUNA SAUCE

CHO 70g/kcalories 660
Serves 3–4

Metric/Imperial		American
1 x 15ml sp/ 1 tbs	olive oil	1 tbs
2	cloves garlic, crushed	2
2–3	sticks celery, chopped	2–3
1	bay leaf	1
pinch	oregano	pinch
	salt and freshly ground black pepper	
200g/1 x 7oz	can tuna fish in brine, drained and flaked	¾ cup
400g/1 x 14oz	can tomatoes	1¾ cups
3 x 15ml sp/ 3 tbs	tomato purée	3 tbs

1. Heat the oil in a pan and fry the garlic and celery. Add the herbs and seasoning to taste with salt and freshly ground black pepper. Stir in the tuna fish, tomatoes and tomato purée. Bring to the boil and simmer gently for 20–30 minutes.
2. Meanwhile cook the pasta in plenty of boiling salted water. Serve the tuna sauce as soon as it is ready on a bed of *al dente* pasta accompanied by salad.

Note to Cooks

Remember to take into account the CHO values of any spaghetti: 45g cooked weight of wholemeal spaghetti = 10g CHO.

BAKED FISH

CHO 10g/kcalories 850
Serves 4

Metric/Imperial		American
4	cod steaks	4
3 x 15ml sp/ 3 tbs	olive or sunflower oil	3 tbs
2	cloves garlic, finely sliced	2
4 x 15ml sp/ 4 tbs	fresh parsley, finely chopped	4 tbs
450g/1 lb	tomatoes, deseeded and finely chopped	1 lb
	salt and freshly ground black pepper	
2 x 15ml sp/ 2 tbs	wholemeal breadcrumbs, toasted	2 tbs

1. Arrange the fish in a lightly oiled baking dish.
2. Meanwhile, lightly beat together all other ingredients, apart from the breadcrumbs. Spread some of the mixture over each slice of fish, sprinkle with the breadcrumbs and bake at 375°F/190°C/gas mark 5 for 30–40 minutes, basting occasionally, until crisp on top.
3. Serve with julienne vegetables and new potatoes.

SMOKED HADDOCK PLAIT

CHO 110g/kcalories 1380
Serves 4–6

Metric/Imperial		*American*
25g/1oz	low-fat spread	2 tbs
1	onion, peeled and chopped	1
25g/1oz	flour	¼cup
275ml/½ pint	skimmed milk	1⅓ cups
	salt and freshly ground black pepper	
1 x 15ml sp/ 1 tbs	lemon juice	1 tbs
225g/8oz	smoked haddock, cooked and flaked	1 cup
50g/2oz	sweetcorn	⅓ cup
215g/7oz	puff pastry	½ lb
1	hard-boiled egg, sliced a little beaten egg to glaze	1

1. Heat the low-fat spread in a pan and sauté the onion. Add the flour and milk and stir continuously, until the sauce has thickened. Season to taste with salt and freshly ground black pepper. Add the lemon juice, fish and sweetcorn.

2. Roll the pastry out into an oblong shape 20 by 30cm (8 by 12 inches) and spoon the filling down the centre third of the pastry, layering it with the eggs.

3. Cut the pastry diagonally at 2cm (1 inch) intervals down each side of the oblong. Fold down the top and

Fish

take one strip from each side of the pastry and cross them over the fish. Continue in this way to form a plait. Brush with the beaten egg and bake at 400°F/200°C/gas mark 6 for approximately 25 minutes, or until the pastry is golden brown.

4. Serve with salad.

PRAWN AND CASHEW NUT CURRY

CHO 20g/kcalories 930
Serves 4

Metric/Imperial		American
1 x 15ml sp/ 1 tbs	corn or sunflower oil	1 tbs
1 large	onion, peeled and chopped	1 large
1–2	cloves garlic, crushed	1–2
1.5cm/½ inch piece	fresh root ginger, peeled and finely chopped	½ inch piece
2 x 5ml sp/2 tsp	ground coriander	2 tsp
2 x 5ml sp/2 tsp	paprika	2 tsp
2 x 5ml sp/2 tsp	ground cumin	2 tsp
400g/1 x 14oz	can chopped tomatoes	1¾ cups
350g/12oz	frozen prawns, thawed	3 cups
50g/2oz	unsalted cashew nuts, lightly toasted and chopped	3½ tbs
150g/1 x 5fl oz	carton low-fat natural yogurt	⅔ cup
	salt and freshly ground black pepper	

1. Heat the oil in a pan and gently fry the onion, garlic and ginger. Add the spices and fry for about a minute.
2. Add the chopped tomatoes, prawns and nuts and stir together well. Stir in the yogurt and seasonings and heat gently for about 5 minutes. Serve immediately with rice.

Note to Cooks

Remember to take into account the CHO values of any rice – 3 tbs/3 x 15ml spoonfuls = 10g CHO.

PAPRIKA FISH

CHO 40g/kcalories 920
Serves 4

Metric/Imperial		American
1 x 15ml sp/ 1 tbs	corn or sunflower oil	1 tbs
2	onions, peeled and sliced	2
2 medium-size	potatoes, peeled and cut into 2cm/¾ inch dice	2 medium-size
1	green pepper, deseeded and cut into strips	1
1	red pepper, deseeded and cut into strips	1
1–2 x 15ml sp/ 1–2 tbs	paprika	1–2 tbs
	salt and freshly ground black pepper	
about 210ml/7fl oz	water	¾ cup
675g/1½ lb	haddock fillet, cut into strips	1½ lb

1. Heat the oil in a pan, add the onion and potato and cook over a low heat, stirring frequently, for 5 minutes. Add the peppers and paprika and season with salt and freshly ground black pepper. Mix in the water and simmer over a low heat for approximately 20 minutes until the vegetables are tender.

2. Add the fish and simmer for a further 5–6 minutes until the fish is just cooked. Serve immediately with more potatoes and vegetables.

FISH-STUFFED BAKED POTATOES

CHO 230g/kcalories 1170
Serves 4

Metric/Imperial		American
4 medium-sized	baking potatoes, washed	4 medium-sized
225g/8oz	white fish	½ lb
100g/4oz	skimmed-milk cheese or low-fat cheese	½ cup
1	clove garlic, crushed	1
1 x 15ml sp/ 1 tbs	fresh chives, finely chopped	1 tbs
	salt and freshly ground black pepper	

1. Bake the potatoes at 400°F/200°C/gas mark 6 for approximately 1 hour or until potatoes are tender.
2. Meanwhile, steam the fish for about 6 minutes until just tender and flake it into a bowl, removing any bones and skin. When the potatoes are cooked, cut a slice off the top of each potato and scoop out the flesh into a bowl. Mash it with the cheese and garlic. Fold in the fish and chives and season to taste with salt and freshly ground black pepper.
3. Fill each potato shell with the mixture and bake them at 350°F/180°C/gas mark 4 for 10–15 minutes or until the filling has heated through. Serve immediately with salad.

Fish

MACKEREL WITH LIME

CHO neg/kcalories 2060
Serves 4

Metric/Imperial		American
4	mackerel (each about 225g/8oz), gutted and filleted	4
2	limes, peeled and sliced	2
bunch	spring onions, chopped	bunch
	salt and freshly ground black pepper	
150ml/¼ pint	dry cider	⅔ cup
2	bay leaves	2

1. Put the mackerel in a lightly greased baking dish. Arrange the lime slices and spring onions down the middle of each fish and season with salt and freshly ground black pepper. Close each fish up and secure with wooden cocktail sticks. Pour the cider over them and add the bay leaves.
2. Cover and cook at 350°F/180°C/gas mark 4 for 30–40 minutes or until tender. Serve hot with vegetables and potatoes.

KEDGEREE

CHO 70g/kcalories 1170
Serves 4

Metric/Imperial		American
450g/1 lb	smoked haddock	1 lb
150ml/¼ pint	skimmed milk	⅔ cup
175g/6oz	brown rice, cooked	1 cup
2	size 3 eggs, hard-boiled	2
175g/6oz	frozen peas, cooked	1 cup
	salt and freshly ground black pepper	
	fresh parsley, chopped, to garnish	

1. Poach the fish in the milk for 10–12 minutes or until tender. Drain, reserving the liquor. Remove any skin from the fish and flake the flesh.
2. Add the fish and rice to a pan. Stir in the egg, and a little of the fish liquor. Add peas and season to taste with salt and freshly ground black pepper, then cook gently over a low heat until heated through.
3. Serve immediately, garnished with the parsley.

SAILOR'S PIE

CHO 100g/kcalories 940
Serves 4

Metric/Imperial		American
1 x 15ml sp/	corn or sunflower oil	1 tbs
1 tbs		
1	onion, peeled and sliced	1
2	sticks celery, sliced	2
50g/2oz	button mushrooms, sliced	¾ cup
3	tomatoes, sliced	3
	salt and freshly ground	
	black pepper	
350g/12oz	white fish, cooked and flaked	2 cups
2–3 drops	Tabasco sauce	2–3 drops
225g/8oz	potatoes, parboiled and	3 cups
	sliced	

1. Heat the oil in a pan and sauté the onion and celery for 2–3 minutes. Add the mushrooms and tomatoes and cook for 3–4 minutes. Put half the mixture in an oven-proof casserole.

2. Season the fish to taste with salt and freshly ground black pepper and put it into the casserole, mixing it in together with the Tabasco sauce. Top with the remaining vegetables.

3. Arrange the sliced potatoes in overlapping circles on top of the casserole and lay a piece of dampened greaseproof paper over them. Cover with foil and bake at 350°F/180°C/gas mark 4 for approximately 1

Diabetes

hour. Then remove the foil and paper and cook under a grill for 2–3 minutes to brown the potatoes. Serve immediately.

HADDOCK CRUMBLE

CHO 100g/kcalories 1100
Serves 4

Metric/Imperial		American
450g/1 lb	haddock	1 lb
275ml/½ pint	skimmed milk	1⅓ cups
1 x 15ml sp/ 1 tbs	corn or sunflower oil	1 tbs
1	onion, peeled and chopped	1
2 x 5ml sp/2 tsp	curry powder	2 tsp
25g/1oz	flour	¼ cup
1 x 15ml sp/ 1 tbs	sultanas	1 tbs
1 x 15ml sp/ 1 tbs	mango chutney	1 tbs
50g/2oz	frozen sweetcorn, cooked salt and freshly ground black pepper	⅓ cup

Crumble topping

25g/1oz	porridge oats	¼ cup
25g/1oz	wholemeal flour	¼ cup
25g/1oz	low-fat spread	2 tbs
1 x 15ml sp/ 1 tbs	fresh parsley, chopped	1 tbs
	salt and freshly ground black pepper	

1. Put the fish and milk in a pan and poach for 10–15 minutes, then drain off the liquid and reserve it. Flake the fish, removing any bones or skin, and put it in a lightly greased ovenproof dish.
2. Heat the oil in a pan and sauté the onion. Stir in the curry powder and flour and cook, stirring, for 1 minute. Stir in the milk and bring to the boil, stirring until it is thick and smooth. Add the sultanas, chutney and sweetcorn. Season to taste with salt and freshly ground black pepper, then pour the sauce over the fish.
3. To make the topping, put the oats and flour in a bowl. Rub in the low-fat spread, then stir in the parsley and seasoning. Spoon it evenly over the fish and cook in the oven at 350°F/180°C/gas mark 4 for 40 minutes. Serve immediately.

STEAMED TROUT WITH
YOGURT SAUCE

CHO 10g/kcalories 750
Serves 4

Metric/Imperial		*American*
4	trout (each about 175g/ 6oz), gutted and cleaned	4
4 x 15ml sp/ 4 tbs	lemon juice	4 tbs
1 x 15ml sp/ 1 tbs	fresh parsley, chopped	1 tbs
	freshly ground black pepper	

Yogurt sauce

1 x 150g/5fl oz	carton low-fat natural yogurt	⅔ cup
1 x 15ml sp/ 1 tbs	horseradish sauce	1 tbs
2 x 15ml sp/ 2 tbs	lemon juice	2 tbs
1–2 x 5ml sp/ 1–2 tsp	fresh chives, chopped	1–2 tsp
pinch	cayenne pepper	pinch

1. Put the trout on a large sheet of foil and season with the lemon juice, parsley and pepper. Fold the foil loosely round the fish to form a parcel and steam for 10 to 15 minutes, or until fish flakes easily when tested with a fork.
2. Meanwhile, to make the sauce, put all the ingredients

in a heatproof bowl. Put it over a pan of simmering water and stir until it is hot and creamy. Remove the trout from the boil and serve immediately with the yogurt sauce poured over them accompanied by julienne vegetables and new potatoes.

STUFFED PLAICE

CHO 40g/kcalories 1450
Serves 4

Metric/Imperial		*American*
8 medium	plaice fillets, skinned	8 medium
3 x 15ml sp/ 3 tbs	unsweetened apple juice	3 tbs
1 x 15ml sp/ 1 tbs	soy sauce	1 tbs

Stuffing

50g/2oz	fresh wholemeal breadcrumbs	1 cup
1–2	cloves garlic, crushed	1–2
1 small	onion, peeled and finely chopped	1 small
25g/1oz	ground almonds	¼ cup
1 x 2.5ml sp/ ½ tsp	ground ginger	½ tsp
2 x 15ml sp/ 2 tbs	unsweetened apple juice	2 tbs
1 x 15ml sp/ 1 tbs	soy sauce	1 tbs
	freshly ground black pepper	

1. Lay the fillets flesh-side down on a clean surface.
2. To make the stuffing, put all the ingredients in a bowl and mix them together well. Divide the stuffing between the fillets and roll up, securing them with

cocktail sticks. Put the rolls in a shallow, lightly greased ovenproof dish.

3. Mix together the apple juice and soy sauce and pour this over the rolled fish. Cover with foil and cook at 350°F/180°C/gas mark 4 for 30 minutes. Serve immediately with vegetables and new potatoes.

HADDOCK AND VEGETABLE CASSEROLE

CHO 40g/kcalories 720
Serves 4

Metric/Imperial		American
1 x 15ml sp/ 1 tbs	corn or sunflower oil	1 tbs
1	onion, peeled and sliced	1
1	green pepper, deseeded and chopped	1
3	tomatoes, chopped	3
1 x 5ml sp/1 tsp	oregano	1 tsp
225g/8oz	potatoes, peeled and cubed	1⅓ cups
1 x 15ml sp/ 1 tbs	tomato purée	1 tbs
	salt and freshly ground black pepper	
450g/1 lb	haddock fillet, skinned and cut into large pieces	1 lb
3 x 15ml sp/ 3 tbs	lemon juice	3 tbs
2	courgettes, sliced	2

1. Heat the oil in a pan and sauté the onion and pepper for 2–3 minutes. Add the tomatoes, oregano, potatoes, tomato purée and season to taste with salt and freshly ground black pepper. Bring to the boil, cover and simmer for 20 minutes, until the potatoes are just tender.

2. Meanwhile, put the fish and lemon juice in a bowl and season. Mix them together well, then add them to the pan, along with the courgettes, cover and simmer for 10 minutes until the fish is tender. Serve immediately with jacket potatoes.

BAKED FISH WITH PEPPER SAUCE

CHO neg/kcalories 1070
Serves 4

Metric/Imperial		American
4	cod or haddock fillets (each about 175g/6oz)	4
25g/1oz	low-fat spread, melted	2 tbs
4 x 15ml sp/ 4 tbs	lemon juice	4 tbs
	salt and freshly ground black pepper	

Pepper sauce

1 x 15ml sp/ 1 tbs	corn or sunflower oil	1 tbs
2	red peppers, deseeded and chopped	2
1 small	onion, peeled and chopped	1 small
2 x 15ml sp/ 2 tbs	half-fat creme fraiche	2 tbs
	lemon twists to garnish	

1. Put the fish in a lightly greased baking dish and brush with the melted low-fat spread. Drizzle with the lemon juice and season to taste with salt and freshly ground black pepper. Cover with foil and cook at 350°F/180°C/gas mark 4 for 20–25 minutes, until tender.

2. Meanwhile, make the sauce. Heat the oil, add the pepper and onion and cook for 5 minutes. Add 3 tbs of water, bring to the boil, cover and cook gently for 10–15 minutes. Transfer the sauce to a blender and process until smooth. Return it to the pan, stir in the creme fraiche and season to taste. Reheat it gently, then serve the fish on warmed serving plates and with the sauce, garnished with the lemon twists and accompanied by vegetables and potatoes.

RICE WITH PRAWNS

CHO 140g/kcalories 1110
Serves 6

Metric/Imperial		American
2 x 15ml sp/ 2 tbs	corn or sunflower oil	2 tbs
1	onion, peeled and chopped	1
1	clove garlic, crushed	1
1 x 5ml sp/1 tsp	ground coriander	1 tsp
1 x 5ml sp/1 tsp	ground cumin	1 tsp
1 x 5ml sp/1 tsp	curry powder	1 tsp
175g/6oz	frozen prawns, thawed	1½ cups
1 x 15ml sp/ 1 tbs	soy sauce	1 tbs
100g/4oz	frozen peas, cooked	⅔ cup
	salt and freshly ground black pepper	
175g/6oz	brown rice, cooked	1 cup
3	spring onions, chopped	3

1. Heat the oil, add the onion and garlic and fry until they have softened. Add the coriander, cumin and curry powder and stir until they are well combined. Stir in the prawns until they are coated in the spices. Add the soy sauce, peas, 4 tbs of water and season to taste with salt and freshly ground black pepper. Cook the mixture for 2 minutes, then add the rice and mix everything together thoroughly. Cover and cook gently until it has heated through.

2. Turn the mixture onto a warmed serving dish, sprinkle the spring onions over it and serve immediately.

MACKEREL WITH MUSTARD AND OATS

CHO 10g/kcalories 1650
Serves 4

Metric/Imperial		*American*
4	mackerel fillets (each about 175g/6oz)	4
1 x 15ml sp/ 1 tbs	lemon juice	1 tbs
	salt and freshly ground black pepper	
2 x 5ml sp/2 tsp	made mustard	2 tsp
25g/1oz	porridge oats	¼ cup

1. Put the mackerel on a grill rack lined with foil. Drizzle the lemon juice over the fish and season with salt and freshly ground black pepper.
2. Stir the mustard and oats together and spread the mixture over the mackerel. Cook the fish under a medium-hot grill for 10–15 minutes, then serve immediately with vegetables and potatoes.

FISH CREOLE

CHO neg/kcalories 560
Serves 4

Metric/Imperial		American
1	onion, peeled and chopped	1
1	green pepper, deseeded and chopped	1
1 x 400g/14oz	can chopped tomatoes	1¾ cups
pinch	basil	pinch
pinch	oregano	pinch
	salt and freshly ground black pepper	
225g/8oz	white fish, cut into cubes	1⅓ cups
225g/8oz	frozen prawns, defrosted	2 cups
1 x 5ml sp/1 tsp	cornflour	1 tsp
2 x 15ml sp/ 2 tbs	dry white wine	2 tbs
	fresh parsley, chopped, to garnish	

1. Put the onion, pepper, tomatoes and herbs and seasoning in a pan and bring to the boil. Cover and simmer for 10 minutes. Add the fish and prawns and simmer for a further 10–15 minutes.
2. Blend the cornflour with the wine, then stir this mixture into the sauce and stir for 1–2 minutes while it thickens. Serve immediately, garnished with the chopped parsley, accompanied by vegetables and potatoes.

Fish

FISH STEAKS AND PEPPERCORN SAUCE

CHO 30g/kcalories 940
Serves 6

Metric/Imperial		American
6	white fish steaks or cutlets	6
25g/1oz	flour	¼ cup
	salt and freshly ground	
	black pepper	

Peppercorn sauce

2 x 15ml sp/ 2 tbs	corn or sunflower oil	2 tbs
150ml/¼ pint	red wine	⅔ cup
150ml/¼ pint	fish stock	⅔ cup
1 x 150ml/ 5fl oz	carton half-fat creme fraiche	⅔ cup
2	tomatoes, chopped	2
2 x 5ml sp/2 tsp	peppercorns, crushed	2 tsp

1. Coat the fish with the flour, to which salt and pepper have been added. Heat the oil in a frying pan and cook the fish for about 5 minutes on each side until it is just tender. Remove the fish to a heated serving dish and keep it warm.

2. Add the wine to the juices in the pan, scraping the pan to ensure that all the sediment is incorporated into the sauce. Boil until the wine has reduced to 3 tbs. Add the stock, stir well and boil until it has reduced to half the original quantity. Add the creme fraiche and stir

over a low heat (do not boil or the creme fraiche will curdle) until the sauce is smooth. Add the tomatoes and peppercorns and adjust the seasoning if necessary. Heat until the sauce is just about to boil, then pour it over the fish and serve immediately with vegetables and potatoes.

SUMMER FISH

CHO neg/kcalories 1030
Serves 4

Metric/Imperial		*American*
	salt and freshly ground black pepper	
4	white fish fillets	4
4 rashers	lean streaky bacon	4 slices
3	courgettes, sliced	3
pinch	dried tarragon	pinch
3 x 15ml sp/ 3 tbs	dry vermouth	3 tbs
150ml/5fl oz carton	half-fat creme fraiche	⅔ cup

1. Season the fish with salt and freshly ground black pepper and wrap a bacon rasher around each fillet, then put them in a lightly greased baking dish. Arrange the courgettes around the fish and sprinkle the tarragon over them.
2. Mix the vermouth and creme fraiche together and pour it over the fish.
3. Cover the dish and bake at 350°F/180°F/gas mark 4 for 20 minutes or until the fish is tender.
4. Serve with vegetables and rice.

STEAMED FISH AND VEGETABLES

CHO neg/kcalories 1200
Serves 6

Metric/Imperial		American
1 x 15ml sp/ 1 tbs	olive or sunflower oil	1 tbs
1	onion, sliced	1
4	carrots, cut into julienne strips	4
3	sticks celery, cut into thin strips	3
1	bulb fennel, cut into thin strips	1
150ml/¼ pint	dry white wine	⅔ cup
150ml/¼ pint	fish stock	⅔ cup
pinch	mixed herbs	pinch
	salt and freshly ground black pepper	
approx. 900g/2 lb	halibut on the bone	2 lb

1. Heat the oil in a shallow pan large enough to accommodate the fish and that has a tight-fitting lid. Add the onion, carrots, celery and fennel and cook for 2–3 minutes. Add the wine and bring it to the boil for 3 minutes to reduce it. Then add the stock, herbs and seasonings. Put the fish on top of the vegetables, cover and steam it over a low heat for about 20 minutes until the fish is cooked.

Fish

2. Remove the fish, put the vegetables onto a warmed serving dish and place the fish on top. Pour the sauce over the fish and serve immediately with potatoes.

SALMON PARCELS

CHO neg/kcalories 850
Serves 4

Metric/Imperial		American
4	salmon steaks	4
25g/1oz	low-fat spread	2 tbs
4	bay leaves	4
4	sprigs parsley	4
1	onion, quartered	1
4 slices	lemon	4 slices
	salt and freshly ground black pepper	

1. Put each salmon steak on a square of foil and dot each one with the low-fat spread. Top with a bay leaf, a sprig of parsley, quarter of onion, slice of lemon and seasonings.
2. Wrap the steaks in the foil and put the parcels in an ovenproof dish. Barely cover the bottom of the dish with water and bake at 350°F/180°C/gas mark 4 for 15–20 minutes or until the salmon is tender. Serve immediately with new potatoes and vegetables.

FISH CAKES

CHO 60g/kcalories 550
Makes 4

Metric/Imperial		*American*
225g/8oz	smoked haddock, cooked and flaked	1⅓ cups
225g/8oz	potatoes, boiled and mashed	1 cup
1 x 15ml sp/ 1 tbs	fresh parsley, chopped	1 tbs
1 x 5ml sp/1 tsp	lemon juice	1 tsp
	salt and freshly ground black pepper	
	a little olive or sunflower oil for frying	

Coating

1	size 3 egg, beaten	1
50g/2oz	wholemeal breadcrumbs	½ cup

1. In a bowl, mix the fish, potatoes, parsley, lemon juice and salt and pepper, binding them together with 1 tbs milk if needed. Shape them into 4 cakes and dip them in the beaten egg, then coat them in the breadcrumbs.
2. Heat the oil (about 3 tbs should be enough) and fry the fish cakes for 5–7 minutes on each side or until they are golden brown then serve with baked beans.

7

Vegetarian Dishes

VEGETARIAN MEALS generally contain more protein and fibre than meat or fish-based meals. They are often more colourful and have a wonderful texture. They are more economical too. Pasta, rice, beans and other pulses are ideal for fast meals as they are quick to prepare and very versatile when combined with different sauces or fillings.

Whether you are vegetarian or not, the recipes in this section are tasty and offer imaginative ways of eating healthily.

PASTA AND PESTO SAUCE

CHO 150g/kcalories 2210
Serves 4

Metric/Imperial		*American*
75g/3oz or 5 x 15ml sp/ 5 tbs	fresh basil	5 tbs
50g/2oz	pine nuts	⅓ cup
2–3	cloves garlic, crushed	2–3
1 x 1.25ml sp/ ¼ tsp	salt	¼ tsp
	freshly ground black pepper	
150ml/¼ pint	olive or rapeseed oil	⅔ cup
2 x 15ml sp/ 2 tbs	Parmesan cheese, finely grated	2 tbs
175g–225g/ 6–8oz	wholewheat pasta, cooked	½ lb

1. Put the basil, pine nuts, garlic and salt in a blender or food processor and blend for 1–2 minutes.
2. Slowly add the oil, a little at a time, then stir in the cheese by hand.
3. Toss it well with the freshly cooked *al dente* pasta.

VEGETABLE LASAGNE

CHO 40g/kcalories 1120
Serves 4–6

Metric/Imperial		*American*
Filling		
1 x 15ml sp/ 1 tbs	olive or sunflower oil	1 tbs
1	onion, sliced	1
1	clove garlic, crushed	1
1	green pepper, deseeded and chopped	1
2 medium	carrots, peeled and thinly sliced	2 medium
100g/4oz	button mushrooms, sliced	1½ cups
1 x 400g/14oz	can tomatoes	1¾ cups
1 x 5ml sp/1 tsp	mixed herbs	1 tsp
	salt and freshly ground black pepper	
225g/8oz	frozen spinach, defrosted and drained	1 cup
6 slices	pre-cooked lasagne	6 slices
White sauce		
15g/½oz	polyunsaturated margarine	1 tbs
15g/½oz	wholemeal flour	1 tbs
150ml/¼ pint	skimmed milk	⅔ cup
25g/1oz	reduced-fat or vegetarian cheddar cheese, grated	¼ cup

Topping

25g/1oz	reduced-fat cheddar cheese, grated	¼ cup
25g/1oz	unsalted cashew nuts	2 tbs

1. Heat the oil in a pan and lightly sauté the onion and garlic in the oil. Add the pepper, carrot and mushrooms and cook for about 5 minutes. Stir in the tomatoes, herbs and season to taste with salt and freshly ground black pepper. Allow to simmer for 5–10 minutes, stirring occasionally.
2. Meanwhile, make the white sauce. Melt the margarine, stir in the flour and cook for 1 minute. Gradually stir in the milk and bring to the boil, stirring continuously until the sauce has thickened. Stir in the cheese and season to taste.
3. Layer the bolognese mixture, with the spinach and lasagne sheets in alternate layers in an oblong dish, ending with a layer of lasagne. Cover the top with the cheese sauce and sprinkle with the cashew nuts and the remaining cheese. Bake at 350°F/180°C/gas mark 4 for 30–35 minutes.
4. Serve with salad.

RED LENTIL LASAGNE

CHO 220g/kcalories 1800
Serves 6

Metric/Imperial		American
225g/8oz	red lentils	1 cup
1 x 15ml sp/ 1 tbs	olive or sunflower oil	1 tbs
1 large	onion, chopped	1 large
2	cloves garlic, crushed	2
1	green pepper, deseeded and chopped	1
100g/4oz	mushrooms, sliced	1½ cups
1 x 5ml sp/1 tsp	dried basil	1 tsp
1 x 5ml sp/1 tsp	dried oregano	1 tsp
1 x 400g/14oz	can chopped tomatoes	1¾ cups
1 x 5ml sp/1 tsp	yeast extract	1 tsp
275ml/½ pint	water	1⅓ cups
1	bay leaf	1
	salt and freshly ground black pepper	
8 sheets	pre-cooked spinach lasagne (lasagne verde)	8 sheets

White sauce

25g/1oz	low-fat spread	2 tbs
25g/1oz	wholemeal flour	¼ cup
275ml/½ pint	skimmed milk	1⅓ cups
1 x 5ml sp/1 tsp	mustard powder	1 tsp
	salt and freshly ground black pepper	

Vegetarian Dishes

| 75g/3oz | reduced-fat vegetarian cheese, grated | ¾ cup |

1. Bring the lentils to the boil in plenty of unsalted water. Boil them fast for 10 minutes, then drain them.
2. Heat the oil in a pan and gently fry the onion and garlic over a moderate heat for 5 minutes. Add the pepper and mushrooms and cook for 5 minutes, stirring from time to time.
3. Add the basil, oregano and drained lentils and cook gently for 2–3 minutes. Stir in the tomatoes and their juice, the yeast extract, water and bay leaf. Bring to the boil, cover and simmer for 15–20 minutes until the lentils are soft. Season with salt and freshly ground black pepper, then remove the bay leaf.
4. Next, make the white sauce. Melt the low-fat spread in a small pan and stir in the flour. Cook it over a gentle heat from 2–3 minutes, stirring. Remove the pan from the heat and gradually stir in the milk. Bring to the boil, stirring all the time, until the sauce thickens. Cook gently for 1–2 minutes. Remove the pan from the heat and beat in the mustard powder and seasoning and a third of the cheese.
5. In a rectangular dish, layer the lentil sauce and lasagne sheets, finishing with a layer of lasagne. Pour the cheese sauce over the top and sprinkle the remaining cheese over it.
6. Bake the lasagne in the oven at 350°F/180°C/gas mark 4 for 30–35 minutes until the cheese has melted, is bubbling and golden brown.

Diabetes

VEGETARIAN PAELLA

CHO 40g/kcalories 630
Serves 2–4

Metric/Imperial		American
1 x 15ml sp/ 1 tbs	olive or sunflower oil	1 tbs
2	onions, peeled and chopped	2
2	cloves of garlic, crushed	2
100g/4oz	brown rice	½ cup
275ml/½ pint	vegetable stock	1⅓ cups
pinch	dried basil	pinch
2	courgettes, washed and sliced	2
1	red pepper, deseeded and sliced	1
1 x 227g/8oz	can tomatoes	1 cup
	freshly ground black pepper	
50g/2oz	reduced-fat cheddar cheese, grated	1/2 cup
15g/½oz	flaked almonds	2 tbs

1. Heat the oil in a pan and add the onions and garlic. Add the rice and cook for a further few minutes coating the grains well with the oil. Add the stock and basil, bring to the boil, reduce the heat, cover and simmer for 25–30 minutes. Add the courgettes, pepper and tomatoes. Season with black pepper and cook for about 10 minutes until the rice is cooked and the vegetables are tender.

Vegetarian Dishes

2. Spoon the mixture into an ovenproof dish. Sprinkle the cheese and almonds over the top and grill until lightly browned. Serve immediately with salad.

THREE-BEAN CASSOULET

CHO 80g/kcalories 770
Serves 4

Metric/Imperial		*American*
1	onion, peeled and sliced	1
1	clove garlic, crushed	1
1 x 400g/14oz	can flageolet beans, drained	2 cups
1 x 225g/8oz	can red kidney beans, drained and refreshed under cold running water	1¼ cups
100g/4oz	cut green beans, cooked	1 cup
1 x 225g/8oz	can tomatoes	1 cup
pinch	mixed herbs	pinch
	salt and freshly ground black pepper	
150ml/¼ pint	vegetable stock	⅔ cup
25g/1oz	sunflower seeds, toasted	2 tbs

1. Put all the ingredients, except the sunflower seeds, into a flameproof casserole and bring to the boil. Simmer for about 20 minutes, stirring occasionally.
2. Sprinkle the sunflower seeds over the top just before you serve with rice or potatoes.

BEAN AND VEGETABLE STEW

CHO 100g/kcalories 1020
Serves 4–6

Metric/Imperial		*American*
1 x 15ml sp/ 1 tbs	corn or sunflower oil	1 tbs
2	cloves garlic, crushed	2
450g/1 lb	leeks, sliced	1 lb
1 large	carrot, sliced	1 large
225g/8oz	mushrooms, sliced	3 cups
1 x 15ml sp/ 1 tbs	paprika	1 tbs
1 x 15ml sp/ 1 tbs	light soy sauce	1 tbs
275ml/½ pint	vegetable stock	1⅓ cups
1 x 225g/8oz	can red kidney beans, drained and refreshed under cold running water salt and freshly ground black pepper	1¼ cups

Dumplings

100g/4oz	self-raising 100 per cent wholemeal flour	1 cup
50g/2oz	vegetable suet	¼ cup
pinch	salt	pinch
1 x 15ml sp/ 1 tbs	parsley, chopped	1 tbs
	a little water to bind	

1. Heat the oil in a flameproof casserole. Add the garlic, leeks, carrot and mushrooms and sauté them until they are tender. Add the paprika, soy sauce and stock and bring to the boil. Add the kidney beans, salt and freshly ground black pepper and simmer for 20 minutes.

2. Meanwhile, make the dumplings. Mix all the ingredients together to make a firm dough. Shape it into 6–8 dumplings and arrange them on top of the stew. Cover the casserole and simmer gently for 20 minutes until the dumplings are light and fluffy, then serve straight away with potatoes.

CHICKPEA MOUSSAKA

CHO 160g/kcalories 1270
Serves 4

Metric/Imperial		*American*
1 large	aubergine	1 large
350g/12oz	potatoes, peeled	¾ lb
1	onion, peeled and finely chopped	1
2	cloves garlic, crushed	2
1 x 15ml sp/ 1 tbs	olive or sunflower oil	1 tbs
50g/2oz	mushrooms, sliced	¾ cup
1 x 400g/14oz	can chopped tomatoes	1¾ cup
2 x 5ml sp/2 tsp	dried oregano	2 tsp
1 x 15ml sp/ 1 tbs	Worcestershire sauce	1 tbs
dash of	Tabasco sauce	dash of
1 x 400g/14oz	can chick peas, drained sea salt and freshly ground black pepper	2¼ cups

Topping

2	size 3 eggs, beaten	2
1 x 5ml sp/1 tsp	cumin seeds, toasted (optional)	1 tsp
1 x 150ml/ 5fl oz	carton low-fat natural yogurt	⅔ cup
	tomato slices and parsley, to garnish	

Diabetes

1. Prick and trim the aubergines and bake them in a 350°F/180°C/gas mark 4 oven for 20–30 minutes, then slice (leaving the oven on).
2. Boil the potatoes until they are tender, then slice them thickly.
3. Gently fry the onion and garlic in the oil for 4–5 minutes. Add the mushrooms, tomatoes, oregano, Worcestershire and Tabasco sauces, chick peas and season with salt and freshly ground black pepper. Cook gently for 10 minutes, adjusting the seasoning if necessary.
4. Arrange layers of aubergine, potato and vegetable sauce in an ovenproof casserole dish, finishing with a layer of aubergine. Beat together the topping ingredients and spoon the mixture over the moussaka. Bake in the oven for 25–30 minutes.

MIXED BEAN HOT POT

CHO 120g/kcalories 660
Serves 3–4

Metric/Imperial		*American*
1 x 225g/8oz	tin cannellini beans, drained and rinsed	1¼ cups
100g/4oz	French beans	1 cup
1 x 227g/8oz	can tomatoes	1 cup
1 x 15ml sp/ 1 tbs	tomato purée	1 tbs
1	clove garlic, crushed	1
1 x 5ml sp/1 tsp	mixed herbs salt and freshly ground black pepper	1 tsp
225g/8oz	potatoes, parboiled and sliced	2¾ cups
25g/1oz	reduced-fat vegetarian cheddar cheese, grated	¼ cup

1. Mix all the ingredients together, except the potatoes and cheese, and pour into an ovenproof dish. Arrange the sliced potatoes on top of the mixture and sprinkle the cheese over them.
2. Cook at 325°F/170°C/gas mark 3 for 45 minutes–1 hour or until the potatoes are cooked.

BRAISED GREEN LENTILS

CHO 110g/kcalories 990
Serves 4

Metric/Imperial		American
225g/8oz	green lentils	1 cup
1 x 15ml sp/ 1 tbs	olive or sunflower oil	1 tbs
1	onion, peeled and finely chopped	1
1 small	potato, cut into small pieces	1 small
1	carrot, scrubbed and diced	1
1	leek, washed and finely sliced	1
2	tomatoes, seeded and diced	2
275ml/½ pint	vegetable stock	1⅓ cups
1 small	garlic clove, crushed salt and freshly ground black pepper	1 small
1 x 5ml sp/1 tsp	white wine vinegar	1 tsp

1. Wash the lentils thoroughly and leave to drain.
2. Heat the oil in a pan and sauté the remaining vegetables gently, stirring all the time, for about 3–4 minutes. Add the stock, garlic and drained lentils and bring to the boil. Simmer until the lentils are just tender (about 7–10 minutes).
3. Season to taste with salt and freshly ground black pepper and add the vinegar.

Note to Cooks

This mixture can be used to make a vegetarian Shepherd's Pie by piping creamed potato over the top.

LENTIL MOUSSAKA

CHO 150g/kcalories 1310
Serves 6

Metric/Imperial		American
2 medium	aubergines, sliced	2 medium
2 x 15ml sp/ 2 tbs	olive oil	2 tbs
2 medium	onions, peeled and chopped	2 medium
100g/4oz	green lentils, cooked	½ cup
1 x 5ml sp/1 tsp	mixed herbs	1 tsp
1 x 5ml sp/1 tsp	nutmeg, grated	1 tsp
1 x 15ml sp/ 1 tbs	tomato purée	1 tbs
1 x 400g/14oz	can tomatoes, drained and chopped, reserving the juice	1¾ cups
600g/22oz	potatoes, parboiled and sliced	3 cups

White sauce

25g/1oz	low-fat spread	2 tbs
25g/1oz	flour	¼ cups
275ml/½ pint	skimmed milk	1⅛ cups
1	size 3 egg	1
	salt and freshly ground black pepper	
1 x 2.5ml sp/ ½ tsp	nutmeg, grated	½ tsp
1	tomato, sliced	1

1. Sprinkle the aubergine slices with salt and leave to stand for 30 minutes to remove the bitter juices. Pat dry with kitchen paper towels. Then heat the oil in a pan and fry the aubergines until they are golden brown. Set aside.

2. Fry the onions in the pan until they are soft, then add the lentils, herbs, nutmeg, tomato purée and tomato juice. Simmer for 5 minutes.

3. Assemble the moussaka by arranging a layer of aubergine slices in an ovenproof dish, followed by slices of potato, chopped tomatoes and the lentil texture. Repeat until all ingredients are used, ending with a layer of aubergine slices.

4. To make the sauce, melt the low-fat spread in a pan, stir in the flour, then gradually add the milk. Bring to the boil, stirring all the time, then reduce the heat and simmer for 2–3 minutes until the sauce is thickened, stirring continuously. Remove the pan from the heat, season to taste and allow to cool slightly before beating in the egg quickly until the sauce is glossy. Pour the sauce over the moussaka. Garnish with the sliced tomato. Bake at 375°F/190°C/gas mark 5 for 45 minutes and serve hot.

MUNG BEAN AND
VEGETABLE COTTAGE PIE

CHO 190g/kcalories 1220
Serves 4–6

Metric/Imperial		American
2 x 5ml sp/2 tsp	sunflower oil	2 tsp
1	onion, finely chopped	1
2	carrots, finely chopped	2
3 sticks	celery, diced	3 sticks
225g/8oz	mung beans, cooked	1¼ cups
2 x 5ml sp/2 tsp	cayenne pepper	2 tsp
1 x 5ml sp/1 tsp	fresh marjoram, chopped	1 tsp
1 x 5ml sp/1 tsp	fresh sage, chopped	1 tsp
1 x 15ml sp/ 1 tbs	tomato purée	1 tbs
1 x 5ml sp/1 tsp	yeast extract	1 tsp
275ml/½ pint	vegetable stock	1⅓ cups
	salt and freshly ground black pepper	
450g/1 lb	potatoes, peeled and diced	2⅔ cups
4 x 15ml sp/ 4 tbs	skimmed milk	4 tbs
15g/½oz	sunflower seeds	1 tbs

1. Preheat the oven to 350°F/180°C/gas mark 4.
2. Heat the oil in a large pan and fry the onion, carrots and celery for 5 minutes. Add the cooked mung beans, cayenne pepper, herbs, tomato purée, yeast extract and stock. Cover and simmer gently for 10–15 minutes.

Vegetarian Dishes

Season to taste with salt and freshly ground black pepper.

3. Meanwhile, boil the potatoes until they are cooked. Drain and mash them with the milk. Put the bean mixture into a large casserole dish and top this with the mashed potato. Sprinkle the sunflower seeds over the top and bake in the preheated oven for 30–40 minutes, until the top is golden brown.

COURGETTE AND SWEETCORN GRATIN

CHO 110g/kcalories 1100
Serves 4–6

Metric/Imperial		*American*
100g/4oz	red lentils	½ cup
2 x 5ml sp/2 tsp	olive or sunflower oil	2 tsp
1	onion, peeled and finely chopped	1
1	clove garlic, crushed	1
1 x 15ml sp/ 1 tbs	tomato purée	1 tbs
50g/2oz	oatmeal	½ cup
1 x 15ml sp/ 1 tbs	lemon juice	1 tbs
1 x 5ml sp/1 tsp	dried mixed herbs	1 tsp
	salt and freshly ground black pepper	

Filling

100g/4oz	courgettes, finely diced	1 cup
100g/4oz	red pepper, deseeded and finely diced	1 cup
1	size 3 egg, beaten	1
1 x 15ml sp/ 1 tbs	wholemeal flour	1 tbs
100ml/4fl oz	skimmed milk	⅓ cup
100g/4oz	canned sweetcorn	⅔ cup
	salt and freshly ground black pepper	
50g/2oz	vegetarian cheese, grated	½ cup

Vegetarian Dishes

1. Boil the lentils in plenty of unsalted water. Boil them fast for 10 minutes then drain them well.

2. Heat the oil in a pan and gently fry the onion for 2–3 minutes. Add the garlic and fry it for 1 minute. Remove the pan from the heat and mix in the lentils, tomato purée, oatmeal, lemon juice and herbs. Season to taste with salt and freshly ground black pepper. The mixture should be thick enough to hold together, but if the lentils are still a little wet, return the pan to the heat to dry it out a little, stirring, or add a little more oatmeal. Press the mixture around the sides and bottom of a 20cm/8 inch flan dish.

3. For the filling, lightly steam the courgettes and pepper for 4 minutes or until tender. Blend the egg with the flour, then add the milk. Stir in the cooked courgettes and sweetcorn and season well. Spoon the filling into the flan dish, cover the top with the cheese. Bake at 375°F/190°C/gas mark 5 for 30–35 minutes, or until the filling has set and serve hot with jacket potatoes and salad.

STIR-FRIED VEGETABLES

CHO neg/kcalories 400
Serves 4

Metric/Imperial		*American*
1 x 15ml sp/ 1 tbs	olive or sunflower oil	1 tbs
4	carrots, cut into strips	4
½	cauliflower, broken into florets	½
175g/6oz	baby sweetcorn	1 cup
100g/4oz	runner beans, cut into pieces	1 cup
100g/4oz	button mushrooms, sliced	1½ cups
225g/8oz	beansprouts	4 cups
2 x 5ml sp/2 tsp	soy sauce	2 tsp

1. Heat the oil in a wok or large frying pan.
2. Add the carrots, cauliflower, sweetcorn and beans and stir for 1–2 minutes. Add the remaining vegetables and cook 1–2 more minutes. Toss the vegetables in the soy sauce and serve immediately with rice.

VEGETABLE CASSEROLE

CHO 10g/kcalories 190
Serves 4

Metric/Imperial		*American*
1 small	swede (about 225g/8oz), peeled and finely diced	1 small
2	carrots, peeled and sliced	2
1	large onion, peeled and chopped	1
4 sticks	celery, chopped	4 sticks
1 x 400g/14oz	can tomatoes	1¾ cups
	salt and freshly ground black pepper	
pinch	ground nutmeg	pinch
about 150ml/¼ pint	vegetable stock	⅔ cup

1. Mix the prepared vegetables together in a 1.75l/3 pint casserole dish. Season to taste with salt and freshly ground black pepper.
2. Pour the tomatoes and some of the stock over the vegetables and cook at 350°F/180°C/gas mark 4 for 1–1¼ hours, or until the vegetables are tender. Add some extra stock if the mixture begins to get a little dry.
3. Serve with jacket potatoes.

CHEESY LEEK AND POTATO CASSEROLE

CHO 110g/kcalories 930
Serves 4–6

Metric/Imperial		*American*
450g/1 lb	leeks, sliced	1 lb
1	onion, peeled and finely sliced	1
450g/1 lb	potatoes, thickly sliced	1 lb
25g/1oz	low-fat spread	2 tbs
25g/1oz	wholemeal flour	¼ cup
275ml/½ pint	skimmed milk	1⅓ cups
1 x 2.5ml sp/ ½ tsp	mustard	½ tsp
	sea salt	
1 x 2.5ml sp/ ½ tsp	paprika	½ tsp
1 x 2.5ml sp/ ½ tsp	ground cumin	½ tsp
50g/2oz	vegetarian cheese, grated	½ cup
1 x 2.5ml sp/ ½ tsp	cumin seeds (optional)	½ tsp

1. Preheat the oven to 350°F/180°C/gas mark 4.
2. Steam the leeks over a large pan of simmering water for 8 minutes.
3. Meanwhile, cover the potato slices with water, bring to the boil and simmer gently for 8 minutes. Drain well.

4. While the potatoes are cooking, melt the low-fat spread in a pan, add the flour and cook gently, stirring, for 2–3 minutes. Remove the pan from the heat and gradually stir in the milk. Return the pan to the heat, bring the sauce to the boil, stirring constantly, and cook gently for 2–3 minutes. Stir in the mustard, seasoning and spices.

5. Layer the leek, onion and potato slices in a casserole or ovenproof dish. Pour the sauce over them and top with the grated cheese. Sprinkle the cumin seeds over, if using. Bake in the preheated oven for 30 minutes, or until the top is golden brown and the vegetables are cooked.

MIXED VEGETABLE CURRY

CHO 50g/kcalories 470
Serves 4–6

Metric/Imperial		American
2 x 5ml sp/2 tsp	olive or sunflower oil	2 tsp
1 x 5ml sp/1 tsp	cumin seeds	1 tsp
1 x 5ml sp/1 tsp	coriander seeds	1 tsp
1 large	onion, peeled and finely chopped	1 large
3	cloves garlic, crushed	3
1 x 5ml sp/1 tsp	garam masala	1 tsp
1 x 2.5ml sp/ ½ tsp	chilli powder	½ tsp
2 medium	potatoes, finely diced	2 medium
100g/4oz	cauliflower, cut into florets	1 cup
2	courgettes, sliced	2
1	leek, sliced	1
1	green pepper, deseeded and cut into strips	1
25g/1oz	wholemeal flour	¼ cup
1 x 400g/14oz	can chopped tomatoes	1¾ cups
150ml/¼ pint	vegetable stock	⅔ cups
2 x 15ml sp/ 2 tbs	low-fat natural yogurt	2 tbs
	salt and freshly ground black pepper	

1. Heat the oil in a large pan and gently cook the cumin and coriander seeds for 3–4 minutes until the seeds are turning brown.
2. Add the onion, garlic, garam masala and chilli powder and cook gently for 2 minutes.
3. Add the potato, cauliflower, courgette, leek and green pepper and continue cooking for 3 minutes, stirring well to ensure that the vegetables are well coated in spices. Sprinkle the flour over them and cook for 1 minute.
4. Add the tomatoes and their juice together with the stock.
5. Bring to the boil, cover and simmer gently for 40–45 minutes, stirring occasionally, adding a little extra stock if the sauce thickens a little too much.
6. When the vegetables are tender, add the yogurt. Adjust the seasoning to taste and serve hot with rice.

Notes to Cooks

The flavours of the curry will have more time to develop if the dish is made a day in advance. 1–2 tablespoons of curry powder may be used in place of the various spices if you do not have them.

STIR-FRIED VEGETABLE SALAD

CHO neg/kcalories 335
Serves 3

Metric/Imperial		American
1 x 15ml sp/ 1 tbs	olive oil or sunflower oil	1 tbs
1	clove garlic, crushed	1
1 small piece	root ginger, peeled and crushed	1 small piece
1 x 2.5ml sp/ ½ tsp	coriander seed, crushed	½ tsp
1 medium	onion, peeled and chopped	1 medium
100g/4oz	baby sweetcorn, trimmed	1 cup
3 small	courgettes, cut into wedges	3 small
1 small	red pepper, deseeded and sliced	1 small
1 small	green pepper, deseeded and sliced	1 small
	salt and freshly ground black pepper	
1 x 15ml sp/ 1 tbs	light soy sauce	1 tbs
1 x 5ml sp/1 tsp	fresh coriander leaves to garnish	1 tsp

1. Heat the oil in a wok or large frying pan with a close-fitting lid.
2. Add the garlic, ginger and coriander seed and cook for

a minute. Add the onion, sweetcorn and courgettes. Cover and cook for a few minutes.

3. Add the peppers, cover and cook for 5 minutes, stirring occasionally. Season with salt and freshly ground black pepper.

4. Remove the pan from the heat and add the soy sauce. Serve warm, garnished with the fresh coriander leaves, accompanied by rice.

SAVOURY CRUMBLE

CHO 180g/kcalories 1500
Serves 4–6

Metric/Imperial		*American*
2 x 5ml sp/2 tsp	olive or sunflower oil	2 tsp
1	onion, peeled and chopped	1
100g/4oz	mushrooms, sliced	1½ cups
100g/4oz	carrots, sliced	⅔ cup
1 small	cauliflower, cut into florets	1 small
2 x 5ml sp/2 tsp	fresh rosemary, chopped	2 tsp
1 x 15ml sp/ 1 tbs	wholemeal flour	1 tbs
275ml/½ pint	vegetable stock salt and freshly ground black pepper	1⅓ cups
1 x 425g/15oz	can butter beans, drained	2⅓ cups
1 x 225g/8oz	can kidney beans, drained and refreshed under cold running water	1¼ cups

Topping

50g/2oz	porridge or jumbo oats	½ cup
50g/2oz	100 per cent wholemeal flour	½ cup
25g/1oz	hazelnuts, chopped	3 tbs
25g/1oz	low-fat spread	2 tbs

1. Heat the oil in a large frying pan with a close-fitting lid over a moderate heat and fry the onion, mushrooms,

carrots and cauliflower. Cover and cook for 5 minutes, stirring frequently. Then, sprinkle the rosemary and flour over the vegetables and cook for 2–3 minutes.

2. Pour on the stock, bring to the boil and simmer gently for 2 minutes. Add salt and freshly ground black pepper to taste, then the butter and kidney beans. Pour the mixture into a casserole or ovenproof dish.

3. For the topping, mix together the oats, flour, hazelnuts and low-fat spread. Sprinkle it on top of the vegetables and bake at 350°F/180°C/gas mark 4 for 30 minutes. Serve hot.

STUFFED PEPPER

CHO 30g/kcalories 210
Serves 1

Metric/Imperial		*American*
1 medium	green or red pepper	1 medium
1 x 5ml sp/1 tsp	corn or sunflower oil	1 tsp
25g/1oz	brown rice, cooked	1 tbs
25g/1oz	frozen peas	2 tbs
25g/1oz	frozen sweetcorn	2 tbs
1 x 15ml sp/ 1 tbs	raisins	1 tbs
	salt and freshly ground black pepper	

1. Slice the top off the pepper and remove the seeds and any white pith.
2. Put the pepper in a saucepan of water and bring to the boil. Simmer for 10 minutes or until it is tender. Drain and keep it warm.
3. Heat the oil in a saucepan, add the rice, vegetables and raisins and season to taste with salt and freshly ground black pepper. Heat thoroughly, spoon the mixture into the pepper and serve.

NUT ROAST

CHO 60g/kcalories 1220
Makes 6 slices

Metric/Imperial		*American*
1	onion, peeled and finely chopped	1
25g/1oz	low-fat spread	2 tbs
225g/8oz	mixed nuts, chopped	1⅔ cups
100g/4oz	wholemeal breadcrumbs	2 cups
275ml/½ pint	vegetable stock	1⅓ cups
2 x 5ml sp/2 tsp	yeast extract	2 tsp
pinch	mixed herbs	pinch
	salt and freshly ground black pepper	
	slices of tomato to garnish	

1. Sauté the onions until transparent in the low-fat spread that you have melted in a pan.
2. In a large bowl, combine all the other ingredients (reserving 1 tbs of the breadcrumbs) and mix together well. The mixture should be loose.
3. Turn the mixture into a lightly greased 450g/1 lb loaf tin and sprinkle the reserved breadcrumbs over the top. Bake the loaf at 350°F/180°C/gas mark 4 for 30 minutes or until it is golden brown. Allow it to cool before you turn it out, then garnish it with the sliced tomatoes.

BASIC PANCAKE MIXTURE

CHO 130g/kcalories 800
Makes 12

Metric/Imperial		*American*
150g/5oz	plain flour	1¼ cups
pinch	salt	pinch
2	size 3 eggs, lightly beaten	2
275ml/½ pint	skimmed milk	1⅛ cups
150ml/¼ pint	water	⅔ cup
1 x 5ml sp/1 tsp	corn or sunflower oil	1 tsp

1. Sift the flour into a bowl and add a pinch of salt. Make a well in the centre and pour in the eggs.
2. Gradually add the milk and water to the well, stirring round the edge of the well until all the flour becomes amalgamated and smooth. Then mix in the oil and leave to stand for 2–3 hours.
3. When the batter has stood for this time, lightly grease and heat a heavy-bottomed frying pan. Cook approximately 1 tbs of the mixture at a time, spreading it over the pan. Loosen the edges of the pancakes from the pan before tossing. Allow them to cook for 1 minute on each side.

FILLINGS

CHO neg/kcalories 280

Ratatouille Filling

Metric/Imperial		American
1 x 400g/14oz	can chopped tomatoes	1¾ cups
2	onions, peeled and chopped	2
1 small	courgette, sliced	1 small
1	green pepper, deseeded and sliced	1
1–2	cloves garlic, crushed	1–2
pinch	mixed herbs	pinch
	salt and freshly ground black pepper	
50g/2oz	reduced-fat cheddar cheese, grated	½ cup

1. Put all the ingredients except the cheese in a saucepan and simmer for 10–15 minutes, seasoning to taste with salt and freshly ground black pepper.
2. Fill the pancakes with the ratatouille – putting 2–3 tbs of it in the middle of each pancake – then roll them up and put them in an ovenproof dish. Sprinkle the cheese over them and bake for 10 minutes at 350°F/180°C/gas mark 4.

Sweetcorn and Mushroom Filling

Metric/Imperial		American
25g/1oz	low-fat spread	2 tbs
225g/8oz	mushrooms, sliced	3 cups
1 x 300g/11oz	can sweetcorn, drained	1½ cups

Cheese sauce

25g/1oz	low-fat spread	2 tbs
25g/1oz	flour	¼ cup
275ml/½ pint	skimmed milk	1⅓ cups
	salt and freshly ground black pepper	
25g/1oz	reduced-fat cheddar cheese, grated	¼ cup
	salt and freshly ground black pepper	

1. Melt the low-fat spread in a pan, lightly sauté the mushrooms.
2. Meanwhile, make the cheese sauce. Melt the low-fat spread in a pan, stir in the flour and cook for 1 minute. Then lower the heat and gradually add the milk, stirring all the time. Bring the sauce to a boil and stir quickly until the sauce thickens. Add the cheese and stir until it has melted, then add the mushrooms and sweetcorn. Season to taste with salt and freshly ground black pepper.
3. Use to fill the pancakes in the same way as for the Ratatouille filling.

8

Salads and Side Dishes

ACCOMPANIMENTS TO the main course provide colour, texture and a tasty diversion. By using low-fat, high-fibre ingredients, the selection of appetizing recipes in this section gives you all of these and more – health-promoting delicious morsels. Try them on their own, too, for lunches or snacks.

WHOLEWHEAT PASTA SALAD

CHO 40g/kcalories 440
Serves 2

Metric/Imperial		American
50g/2oz	wholewheat pasta, cooked	1 cup
1 medium or 2 small	carrots, sliced	1 medium or 2 small
½	green pepper, deseeded and cut into strips	½
2 stalks	celery, chopped	2 stalks
1 x 2.5ml sp/ ½ tsp	garlic powder	½ tsp
1 x 15ml sp/ 1 tbs	Worcestershire or soy sauce	1 tbs
	fresh parsley, chopped, to garnish	

1. Mix all the ingredients, except the parsley, together in a bowl.
2. Garnish the salad with the chopped parsley.

WALDORF SALAD

CHO 60g/kcalories 570
Serves 4–6

Metric/Imperial		American
3	red apples, diced	3
2 x 15ml sp/ 2 tbs	lemon juice	2 tbs
50g/2oz	walnuts, chopped	½ cup
1 head	celery, chopped	1 head
300g/10fl oz carton	low-fat natural yogurt	1⅓ cups
	a few lettuce leaves to garnish	

1. Put all but a third of the apple in a bowl and drizzle the lemon juice over to prevent it browning. Mix the nuts, celery and natural yogurt with the apple.
2. Arrange the lettuce leaves and salad on a serving dish. Use the reserved apple to garnish the salad.

ITALIAN BEAN SALAD

CHO 50g/kcalories 670
Serves 4

Metric/Imperial		*American*
1 x 425g/15oz	can cannellini beans, drained	2⅓ cups
1 x 200g/7oz	can tuna in brine, drained	1 cup
1 small	onion, peeled and sliced	1 small
4 x 15ml sp/ 4 tbs	Mustard Dressing recipe (see page 175)	4 tbs

1. Put all the ingredients into a bowl and toss together until they are well mixed.
2. Chill in the refrigerator before serving.

RED KIDNEY BEANS WITH WALNUTS

CHO 30g/kcalories 800
Serves 4

Metric/Imperial		American
1 x 227g/8oz	can red kidney beans, drained and refreshed under cold running water	1¼ cups
1 small	fennel bulb, finely chopped	1 small
1	onion, peeled and sliced	1
50g/2oz	walnuts, chopped	½ cup
3 x 15ml sp/ 3 tbs	olive oil	3 tbs
2–3 x 15ml sp/ 2–3 tbs	fresh parsley, chopped	2–3 tbs
2	cloves garlic, crushed salt and freshly ground black pepper	2

1. Mix the kidney beans, fennel, onion and walnuts together in a salad bowl.
2. Season the olive oil with the parsley, garlic and salt and freshly ground black pepper. Dress the vegetable mixture with it and leave to marinate for an hour or so before serving.

AUTUMN SALAD

CHO 40g/kcalories 680
Serves 6

Metric/Imperial		*American*
1	crispy lettuce, shredded	1
1	green pepper, deseeded and sliced	1
2	courgettes, thinly sliced	2
75g/3oz	green lentils, cooked	½ cup
1	Low-calorie French Dressing recipe (see page 174) salt and freshly ground black pepper	1
1 x 5ml sp/1 tsp	ground cumin	1 tsp
50g/2oz	unsalted peanuts, chopped and toasted	½ cup

1. Put the lettuce and green pepper into a salad bowl. Add the courgettes and lentils.
2. Pour the Low-calorie French Dressing over the salad and mix so it coats all the ingredients well. Season to taste with salt and freshly ground black pepper.
3. Just before serving, toss in the chopped peanuts.

RICE SALAD

CHO 145g/kcalories 1095
Serves 6

Metric/Imperial		American
175g/6oz	brown rice, cooked	1 cup
225g/8oz	tomatoes chopped	1 cup
1	green pepper, deseeded and sliced	1
10	green olives, stoned and halved	10
50g/2oz	unsalted peanuts, chopped and toasted	½ cup
1	Low-calorie French Dressing recipe (see page 174) salt and freshly ground black pepper	1

1. Put the rice into a bowl. Add the tomatoes, pepper, olives and peanuts and mix everything together well.
2. Pour in the Low-calorie French Dressing and season to taste with salt and freshly ground black pepper.
3. Chill until you are ready to serve.

RICE AND MILLET SALAD

CHO 160g/kcalories 880
Serves 6–8

Metric/Imperial		American
100g/4oz	long-grained brown rice	½ cup
100g/4oz	millet	½ cup
1	onion, finely chopped	1
6	cardamom pods, slightly crushed	6
20	coriander seeds, crushed	20
pinch	cinnamon	pinch
425ml/¾ pint	vegetable stock	2 cups
2 sprigs	fresh thyme	2 sprigs
	salt and freshly ground black pepper	
4 stalks	celery, trimmed and cut into small chunks	4 stalks
1	red pepper, deseeded and diced	1
25g/1oz	hazelnuts or walnuts, lightly toasted	¼ cup
1 x 15ml sp/ 1 tbs	fresh coriander, roughly chopped	1 tbs

Dressing

1 x 5ml sp/1 tsp	light soy sauce	1 tsp
2 x 15ml sp/ 2 tbs	lemon juice	2 tbs

1. Wash the rice and millet and leave them to drain.
2. Meanwhile, sweat the onion and spices over gentle heat in a non-stick pan for 2–3 minutes. Add the rice and millet, stirring with a wooden spoon, then add the stock and thyme. Stir again to ensure that no grains have stuck to the bottom of the pan and season with salt and freshly ground black pepper. Bring to the boil, cover and simmer for about 20–25 minutes. The grains should now be tender and all the liquid should have been absorbed.
3. Tip the rice and millet into a warmed serving bowl and use a fork to separate the grains, removing the thyme and cardamom pods as you go. Leave it to cool before adding the celery, pepper, nuts and coriander. Mix the dressing and pour it over the salad. Mix everything together well and serve.

PRAWN AND RICE SALAD

CHO 140g/kcalories 1210
Serves 4–6

Metric/Imperial		*American*
175g/6oz	brown rice, cooked	1 cup
225g/8oz	frozen prawns, defrosted	2 cups
4	spring onions, finely chopped	4
1	green pepper, deseeded and chopped	1
2	tomatoes, chopped	2
	salt and freshly ground black pepper	
	fresh parsley, chopped, to garnish	

Dressing

3 x 15ml sp/ 3 tbs	olive oil	3 tbs
1 x 15ml sp/ 1 tbs	lemon juice	1 tbs
pinch	mixed herbs	pinch

1. Put the rice in a bowl.
2. Mix the dressing ingredients in a screw-top jar and pour it over the rice.
3. Add the prawns, spring onions, peppers, tomatoes and seasoning and mix them together well. Serve garnished with the parsley.

Salads and Side Dishes

FISH SALAD PLATTER

CHO neg/kcalories 610
Serves 4

Metric/Imperial		American
225g/8oz	cod fillet, cooked and flaked	1⅓ cups
2 x 15ml sp/ 2 tbs	low-calorie French dressing	2 tbs
2 x 5ml sp/2 tsp	lemon juice	2 tsp
1 x 200g/7oz	can tuna in brine, drained	1 cup
2	size 3 eggs, hard-boiled and quartered	2
	salt and freshly ground black pepper	
1	lettuce, washed	1
3	tomatoes, sliced	3
1	green pepper, deseeded and sliced	1
6	black olives, halved, to garnish	6

1. Put the cod in a bowl. Add the French dressing and lemon juice. Add the tuna and eggs. Toss lightly together and season to taste with salt and freshly ground black pepper.
2. Arrange the lettuce leaves on a platter. Pile the fish mixture on top and arrange the tomato slices and pepper rings around it. Serve garnished with the olives.

FRUIT AND VEGETABLE MIXED SALAD

CHO 90g/kcalories 550
Serves 6–8

Metric/Imperial		*American*
3	carrots, peeled and coarsely grated	3
2	apples, cored and sliced	2
2	pears, cored and sliced	2
6 sticks	celery, finely sliced	6 sticks
½	cucumber, diced	½
50g/2oz	raisins	⅓ cup
1 x 5ml sp/1 tsp	lemon juice	1 tsp
	salt and freshly ground black pepper	
1 x 150g/5fl oz	carton low-fat natural yogurt	⅔ cup

1. Put all the prepared fruit and vegetables into a bowl.
2. Add the lemon juice and seasonings to the yogurt.
3. Mix the yogurt dressing with the salad ingredients and chill well before serving.

SLIMMER'S SALAD

CHO 10g/kcalories 640
Serves 4-6

Metric/Imperial		*American*
450g/1 lb	cottage cheese	2 cups
1 x 150g/	carton low-fat natural	⅔ cup
1 x 5fl oz	yogurt	
2 x 15ml sp/	fresh chives, chopped	2 tbs
2 tbs		
½	cucumber, diced	½
1	red pepper, deseeded and diced	1
½	onion, grated	½
	salt and freshly ground black pepper	
	a few lettuce leaves, shredded, to garnish	

1. Combine the cottage cheese with the yogurt, chives, cucumber, and pepper.
2. Season to taste with the onion, salt and pepper and toss together well.
3. Serve on a bed of the lettuce.

LOW-CALORIE FRENCH DRESSING

CHO neg/kcalories 100
Makes 100ml/4fl oz

Metric/Imperial		*American*
6 x 15ml sp/ 6 tbs	cider or wine vinegar	6 tbs
1 x 15ml sp/ 1 tbs	olive oil	1 tbs
1 x 2.5ml sp/ ½ tsp	dry mustard	½ tsp
	salt and freshly ground black pepper	

1. Measure all the ingredients into a jar with a screw-top lid. Shake them together well and store in the refrigerator until the dressing is needed.
2. Shake the jar vigorously before using as the ingredients settle.

Note to Cooks

This recipe will keep for 2–3 days in the refrigerator.

MUSTARD DRESSING

CHO neg/kcalories 330
Makes 100ml/4fl oz

Metric/Imperial		*American*
3 x 15ml sp/ 3 tbs	olive oil	3 tbs
2 x 15ml sp/ 2 tbs	cider vinegar	2 tbs
1 x 5ml sp/1 tsp	wholegrain mustard	1 tsp
1 small	onion, peeled and grated	1 small
1	clove garlic, crushed	1
pinch	intense sweetener salt and freshly ground black pepper	pinch

1. Measure all the ingredients into a screw-top jar and shake it until well mixed. Chill the dressing in the refrigerator until you need it.
2. Shake the jar well before serving to remix the ingredients as they tend to settle after the initial making.

Note to Cooks

This recipe will keep for 2–3 days in the refrigerator.

TSATZIKI

CHO 20g/kcalories 160
Serves 4–6

Metric/Imperial		American
2 x 150g/5fl oz	cartons, low-fat natural yogurt	⅔ cup
10cm/4 inch piece	cucumber, diced	4 inch piece
1 x 15ml sp/ 1 tbs	fresh mint, chopped	1 tbs
1	clove garlic, crushed (optional)	1
1 sprig	fresh mint to garnish	1 sprig

1. Mix all the ingredients together and chill it well before you serve it.
2. Garnish the Tzatziki with the sprig of mint.

POTATO AND SPROUT BAKE

CHO 80g/kcalories 550
Serves 4-6

Metric/Imperial		*American*
450g/1 lb	potatoes, peeled and diced	2⅔ cups
225g/8oz	Brussels sprouts, peeled and trimmed	2 cups
15g/½ oz	low-fat spread	1 tbs
	freshly grated nutmeg	
	salt and freshly ground black pepper	
25g/1oz	reduced-fat cheddar cheese, grated	¼ cup

1. Cook the potatoes and sprouts·in boiling water for about 15 minutes. Drain, then mash them together with the low-fat spread, nutmeg and season with salt and freshly ground black pepper.
2. Spoon the mixture into a heatproof dish, sprinkle the cheese over the top and grill until the cheese is bubbling and golden brown. Serve immediately.

COOKED CHICORY

CHO neg/kcalories 240
Serves 4

Metric/Imperial		American
50g/2oz	low-fat spread	¼ cup
450g/1 lb	chicory, leaves separated from the stem	1 lb
pinch	salt	pinch
pinch	intense sweetener	pinch
1	lemon, juice of	1

1. Melt the low-fat spread in a pan and toss the chicory leaves in it. Add the salt, sweetener and lemon juice and cover.
2. Cook over a gentle heat for 10 minutes, then serve immediately.

BRAISED CELERY

CHO neg/kcalories 210
Serves 4

Metric/Imperial		*American*
1	onion, peeled and chopped	1
1 medium	carrot, peeled and chopped	1 medium
1	clove garlic, crushed	1
25g/1oz	low-fat spread	2 tbs
2 small	heads of celery, split into individual sticks	2 small
150ml/¼ pint	vegetable stock	⅔ cups
	salt and freshly ground black pepper	
1–2 x 15ml sp/ 1–2 tbs	fresh parsley, chopped	1–2 tbs

1. Lightly sauté the onion, carrot and garlic in the low-fat spread in a pan for 5 minutes. Transfer the vegetables to an ovenproof casserole. Put the celery on top of the vegetables. Pour the stock over it and season well with salt and freshly ground black pepper.
2. Cover and bake at 350°F/180°C/gas mark 4 for approximately 1–1½ hours, turning the celery occasionally in the juices.
3. Serve this dish hot, with the parsley sprinkled over it just before serving.

SPRING CABBAGE

CHO neg/kcalories 360
Serves 4

Metric/Imperial		*American*
25g/1oz	low-fat spread	2 tbs
675g/1½ lb	spring cabbage, shredded	1½ lb
1	onion, peeled and chopped	1
2 rashers	streaky bacon, rind removed and chopped	2 slices
pinch	grated nutmeg	pinch

1. Heat the low-fat spread in a large saucepan, add all the ingredients, cover and cook very gently for 20–30 minutes, until the cabbage is just tender, stirring frequently.
2. Serve immediately.

STUFFED MUSHROOMS

CHO 30g/kcalories 400
Serves 4

Metric/Imperial		*American*
4 large	field mushrooms	4 large
50g/2oz	wholemeal breadcrumbs	1 cup
50g/2oz	reduced-fat cheddar cheese, grated	½ cup
25g/1oz	walnuts, finely chopped	3 tbs
pinch	mixed herbs	pinch
	freshly ground black pepper	
1 x 15ml sp/ 1 tbs	tomato ketchup	1 tbs

1. Remove the mushroom stalks and chop them finely. Mix them together with the remaining ingredients. Spoon equal amounts into each of the mushroom caps and put them on a baking sheet.
2. Bake them at 375°F/190°C/gas mark 5 for 10 minutes. Serve as soon as they are done.

PEPPERS À LA PROVENCE

CHO neg/kcalories 260
Serves 4

Metric/Imperial		American
1 x 15ml sp/ 1 tbs	olive or sunflower oil	1 tbs
2 medium	onions, peeled and sliced	2 medium
1	clove garlic, crushed	1
4	peppers (assorted colours), deseeded and sliced	4
1 x 400g/14oz	can tomatoes	1¾ cups
1 x 5ml sp/1 tsp	*herbs de Provence*	1 tsp
	salt and freshly ground black pepper	

1. Heat the oil in a large pan, add the onions and garlic and fry them until they are soft. Add the peppers and cook for 5–10 minutes.
2. Stir in the tomatoes, herbs and season to taste with salt and freshly ground black pepper. Bring to the boil, then simmer for 15–20 minutes.
3. Serve either hot or cold.

SAUTÉED OKRA

CHO neg/kcalories 180
Serves 4

Metric/Imperial		*American*
1 x 15ml sp/ 1 tbs	olive or sunflower oil	1 tbs
1	onion, peeled and chopped	1
1 x 2.5ml sp/ ½ tsp	chilli powder	½ tsp
1 x 5ml sp/1 tsp	ground coriander	1 tsp
1 x 5ml sp/1 tsp	garam masala	1 tsp
225g/8oz	okra	½ lb
1–2 x 15ml sp/ 1–2 tbs	lemon juice	1–2 tbs
pinch	salt	pinch

1. Heat the oil in a pan and fry the onion, chilli powder, coriander and garam masala. Add the okra and lemon juice and a pinch of salt and cook for approximately 5 minutes.
2. Serve immediately.

STUFFED AUBERGINES

CHO 20g/kcalories 865
Serves 6

Metric/Imperial		American
3 medium	aubergines	3 medium
1 x 15ml sp/ 1 tbs	olive or sunflower oil	1 tbs
2 large	onions, peeled and chopped	2 large
2	cloves garlic, crushed	2
100g/4oz	mushrooms, chopped	1½ cups
4 large	tomatoes, skinned and chopped	4 large
1 x 5ml sp/1 tsp	tomato purée	1 tsp
50g/2oz	wholemeal breadcrumbs	1 cup
2 x 15ml sp/ 2 tbs	bran	2 tbs
25g/1oz	blanched almonds, chopped	3 tbs
1 x 15ml sp/ 1 tbs	fresh parsley, chopped	1 tbs
1 x 5ml sp/1 tsp	lemon juice	1 tsp
	salt and freshly ground black pepper	
50g/2oz	vegetarian cheese, grated	½ cup

1. Pierce the aubergines with a fork to prevent the skins from bursting, put them on a baking tray and bake them for 30 minutes at 350°F/180°C/gas mark 4, turning them once. Cut them in half lengthways and

scoop out the flesh, leaving some to form thick skins for the shells. Chop the flesh.

2. Heat the oil in a pan and fry the onions and garlic over a moderate heat for 2 minutes, stirring occasionally. Add the mushrooms, tomatoes and tomato purée to the pan. Simmer for 5 minutes stirring occasionally, then add the chopped aubergine flesh, two-thirds of the breadcrumbs, half the bran, the almonds, parsley and lemon juice and season to taste with salt and freshly ground black pepper. Stir them all together well and simmer for 2–3 minutes.

3. Put the aubergine shells in an ovenproof dish and spoon the filling into the shells. Mix together the remaining breadcrumbs, bran and the cheese and sprinkle this over the tops of the aubergine shells, pressing down firmly on the filling. Bake for 20–25 minutes, until the cheese is bubbling and golden brown. Serve hot.

LEEKS IN CURRY DRESSING

CHO neg/kcalories 580
Serves 4

Metric/Imperial		*American*
8 medium	leeks, washed and cut into 15cm/5–6 inch lengths and cooked until just tender	8 medium

Dressing

3 x 15ml sp/ 3 tbs	corn or sunflower oil	3 tbs
2 x 15ml sp/ 2 tbs	wine vinegar	2 tbs
1 x 5ml sp/1 tsp	curry powder	1 tsp
1 x 5ml sp/1 tsp	made mustard	1 tsp
	salt and freshly ground black pepper	
pinch	intense sweetener	pinch

1. Arrange the cooled leeks on 4 serving plates.
2. To make the dressing, put all the ingredients in a screw-top jar and shake well.
3. Pour the dressing over the leeks and chill until needed.

COURGETTES À LA GRECQUE

CHO neg/kcalories 330
Serves 4

Metric/Imperial		*American*
2 x 15ml sp/ 2 tbs	olive oil	2 tbs
1	onion, peeled and sliced	1
1–2	cloves garlic, crushed	1–2
450g/1 lb	courgettes, sliced	1 lb
1 x 15ml sp/ 1 tbs	cider vinegar	1 tbs
2 x 15ml sp/ 2 tbs	tomato purée	2 tbs
1 x 5ml sp/1 tsp	thyme	1 tsp
6 x 15ml sp/ 6 tbs	water	6 tbs
	salt and freshly ground black pepper	

1. Heat the oil in a pan and sauté the onion and garlic for 2–3 minutes. Add the courgettes and cook for 5 minutes, stirring occasionally. Add the vinegar, tomato purée, thyme, water and salt and freshly ground black pepper.
2. Mix all the ingredients together well. Bring them to the boil, cover and simmer for 15 minutes. Serve either hot or cold.

MUSHROOMS À LA GRECQUE

CHO neg/kcalories 410
Serves 4

Metric/Imperial		American
2 x 15ml sp/ 2 tbs	olive oil	2 tbs
1	onion, peeled and chopped	1
1	clove garlic, crushed	1
4	tomatoes, skinned, seeded and finely chopped	4
450g/1 lb	button mushrooms, chopped	6 cups
1 x 15ml sp/ 1 tbs	tomato purée	1 tbs
1	wineglass dry white wine	1
2 x 15ml sp/ 2 tbs	fresh parsley, chopped	2 tbs
	salt and freshly ground black pepper	

1. Heat the oil in a pan, add the onion and garlic and fry for 5 minutes. Then add the tomatoes and mushrooms and cook for 5 more minutes, stirring occasionally.
2. Stir in the tomato purée and wine. Bring to the boil then remove the pan from the heat immediately. Add all but 1 tbs of the parsley and season, stir well and leave the mixture to cool.
3. Chill for at least 2 hours before serving. Top with the reserved parsley before serving.

Salads and Side Dishes

SUMMER VEGETABLE SALAD

CHO 20g/kcalories 540
Serves 6

Metric/Imperial		American
2	carrots, sliced	2
100g/4oz	broccoli, cooked *al dente*	1 cup
100g/4oz	French beans, cooked *al dente*	1 cup
100g/4oz	sweetcorn, cooked	⅔ cup
50g/2oz	lentils, cooked	⅓ cup
2	courgettes, thinly sliced	2

Dressing

6 x 15ml sp/ 6 tbs	reduced-calorie mayonnaise	6 tbs
bunch	tarragon, chopped	bunch
2 x 15ml sp/ 2 tbs	lemon juice	2 tbs
	salt and freshly ground black pepper	

1. Put all the vegetables into a salad bowl.
2. Mix all the dressing ingredients together then stir in to the vegetables until they are evenly coated with it. Adjust the seasoning to taste if necessary and chill until needed.

CHEESE AND FRUIT COCKTAIL

CHO 30g/kcalories 300
Serves 4

Metric/Imperial		*American*
2	red-skinned dessert apples, chopped (skins left on)	2
2 sticks	celery, chopped	2 sticks
50g/2oz	reduced-fat cheese, diced	½ cup
50g/2oz	grapes, halved and deseeded	⅓ cup
1	orange, grated zest and juice of	1
2 x 15ml sp/ 2 tbs	low-fat natural yogurt	2 tbs
	a few lettuce leaves, shredded	

1. Put the apples, celery, cheese and grapes into a bowl.
2. Mix the orange juice and yogurt together and add this to the bowl, mixing it together well with the fruit, vegetable and cheese.
3. Arrange the salad on a bed of lettuce and chill until you are ready to serve.

STUFFED ICEBERG LETTUCE

CHO 20g/kcalories 510
Serves 4–6

Metric/Imperial		*American*
1	Iceberg lettuce	1
175g/6oz	skimmed milk or low-fat soft cheese	¾ cup
1 x 15ml sp/ 1 tbs	skimmed milk (if necessary)	1 tbs
1	red pepper, deseeded and finely diced	1
25g/1oz	sultanas	2 tbs
25g/1oz	walnuts, chopped salt and freshly ground black pepper	3 tbs

1. Cut the top off the lettuce and reserve it. Using a sharp knife, scoop out the centre, leaving a 2.5cm/1 inch thick case. Chop the lettuce you scooped out and put it into a bowl.
2. Mix the soft cheese, milk, pepper, sultanas and walnuts together and season to taste with salt and freshly ground black pepper. Add half the chopped lettuce to this mixture and spoon it into the lettuce case and replace the lid.
3. Put the Stuffed Iceberg Lettuce on a serving plate and garnish with the remaining chopped lettuce. Keep it chilled until you are ready to serve.

VEGETABLE RICE

CHO 200g/kcalories 980
Serves 4

Metric/Imperial		American
225g/8oz	long-grain rice	1 cup
100g/4oz	carrots, finely chopped	⅔ cup
100g/4oz	sweetcorn kernels	⅔ cup
1 x 15ml sp/ 1 tbs	parsley, finely chopped	1 tbs

1. Place the rice in a pan of boiling water. Cover and simmer for 15 minutes.
2. Add the vegetables and cook for a further 10 minutes or until the rice is tender.
3. Drain well, stir in the parsley and transfer to a warmed serving dish.

9

Puddings and Desserts

A LMOST EVERYONE loves a good pudding or sophisticated dessert, whether it is hot or cold. What could be a better ending to a meal than a slice of cheesecake or a hearty crumble?

The recipes that follow use fruits that are high in fibre and a good source of vitamins, together with other high-fibre ingredients, such as wholemeal flour and dried fruits, and low-fat ingredients, such as low-fat spreads and dairy products. Where possible the virtually calorie-free artificial sweeteners are used instead of sugar to sweeten a dish and where sugar is used the quantities have been reduced as much as possible. All this means that you can eat a lovely dessert without feeling guilty – as long as you don't get too carried away!

EVE'S PUDDING

CHO 170g/kcalories 1350
Serves 8–10

Metric/Imperial		*American*
450g/1 lb	cooking apples, peeled, cored and sliced	1 lb
1	orange, zest and juice of	1
1	lemon, zest and juice of	1
25g/1oz	hazelnuts, finely chopped	3 tbs
2 x 15ml sp/ 2 tbs	water	2 tbs

Topping

100g/4oz	low-fat spread	½ cup
50g/2oz	caster sugar	⅓ cup
2	size 3 eggs, beaten	2
100g/4oz	wholemeal self-raising flour	1 cup
pinch	baking powder	pinch
pinch	cinnamon	pinch
1 x 15ml sp/ 1 tbs	boiling water	1 tbs

1. Put the sliced apples in a deep 20 by 25cm/8 by 10 inch baking dish. Add the zest and juice of the orange and lemon, the nuts and water and mix them together well. Cover with foil and bake in the oven at 375°F/190°C/ gas mark 5 for 10–12 minutes.
2. Meanwhile, make the topping. Cream the low-fat

spread and sugar together until the texture is light and fluffy. Add the beaten eggs gradually, beating the mixture well between each addition.

3. Gradually add the flour, folding it into the creamed mixture. Add the baking powder, cinnamon and water and mix them into the mixture. Spread the topping evenly over the fruit and return the dish to the oven for a further 25–30 minutes, or until the topping is well risen and springs back when touched. The pudding may be served hot or cold.

BAKED APPLES

CHO 50g/kcalories 190
Serves 2

Metric/Imperial		*American*
2 medium	cooking apples, cores removed	2 medium
25g/1oz	raisins	2 tbs
1 x 2.5ml sp/ ½ tsp	ground cinnamon	½ tsp
1 x 2.5ml sp/ ½ tsp	ground mixed spice	½ tsp

1. Slit the apple skins from top to bottom at intervals and then put them in an ovenproof dish. Mix the raisins with the spices and fill the core of each apple with the fruit mixture.
2. Cover the dish with foil and bake at 350°F/180°C/gas mark 4 for about 30–40 minutes.

BAKEWELL TART

CHO 140g/kcalories 1350
Makes 8–10 portions

Metric/Imperial		American
Pastry		
75g/3oz	wholemeal flour	¾ cup
25g/1oz	plain flour	¼ cup
pinch	salt	pinch
25g/1oz	low-fat spread	2 tbs
25g/1oz	white polyunsaturated vegetable fat	2 tbs
	cold water to mix	
Filling		
2 x 15ml sp/ 2 tbs	pure fruit spread	2 tbs
50g/2oz	low-fat spread	¼ cup
25g/1oz	caster sugar	2 tbs
50g/2oz	ground rice	¼ cup
25g/1oz	ground almonds	¼ cup
1	size 3 egg, beaten	1
few drops	almond essence (optional)	few drops
	blanched almonds to decorate	

1. Make the pastry by sieving the two flours and salt together into a bowl, cutting in the fats until they are well mixed with the flour and then stirring in a little

cold water at a time until the mixture forms a smooth, pliable dough, neither too hard nor too soft. Line an 18cm/7 inch fluted flan ring with the pastry, saving the oddments left over. Spread the pure fruit spread over the bottom.

2. Now make the filling. Cream the low-fat spread and sugar until the mixture becomes light and fluffy. Mix together the ground rice and ground almonds and add this to the creamed mixture with the beaten egg and almond essence (if using), combining all the ingredients together well. Spread the mixture over the jam.

3. Knead the reserved scraps of pastry together, roll it out and cut it into strips. Decorate the top of the tart by making a lattice pattern with the strips and dotting with blanched almonds.

4. Bake the tart at 375°F/190°C/gas mark 5 for 30–35 minutes.

PEACH PUDDING

CHO 130g/kcalories 1120
Serves 10

Metric/Imperial		American
75g/3oz	low-fat spread	⅓ cup
50g/2oz	caster sugar	⅓ cup
2	size 3 eggs, beaten	2
50g/2oz	wholemeal self-raising flour	½ cup
25g/1oz	ground almonds	¼ cup
1 x 5ml sp/1 tsp	ground cinnamon	1 tsp
3	fresh peaches, peeled, stoned and sliced	3
2 x 5ml sp/2 tsp	demerara sugar	2 tsp

1. Cream the low-fat spread and sugar until the mixture has become pale. Beat in the eggs a little at a time alternately with the flour, ground almonds and half the cinnamon. Spoon the mixture into a lightly greased 23cm/9 inch round, shallow ovenproof dish or pie plate. Arrange the peach slices over the mixture and push them into it.

2. Mix the remaining cinnamon with the demerara sugar and sprinkle it over the pudding, then bake it at 375°F/190°C/gas mark 5 for approximately 30 minutes or until it has cooked. The mixture should have risen, be golden brown and the sugar should have caramelized.

Diabetes

204

TRIFLE

CHO 110g/kcalories 1040
Serves 6

Metric/Imperial		*American*
1 x 425g/15oz	can fruit cocktail in natural juice	2 cups
1	packet sugar-free jelly crystals	1
2 x 15ml sp/ 2 tbs	custard powder	2 tbs
275ml/½ pint	skimmed milk intense artificial sweetener to taste	1½ cups
150ml/¼ pint carton	whipping cream, whipped	⅔ cups
	a few flaked almonds, toasted	

1. Drain the fruit and reserve the juice. Arrange the fruit in the bottom of a bowl.
2. Make up the jelly crystals according to the directions on the packet and make up to 550ml/1 pint using the reserved fruit juice. Pour the jelly onto the fruit and leave to set.
3. Make the custard according to the directions on the tin and sweeten if necessary. Pour it over the fruit and top with the whipped cream and toasted almonds.
4. Chill the trifle well before serving.

RASPBERRY AND KIWI WHIP

CHO 40/10g/kcalories 380
Serves 4–6

Metric/Imperial		*American*
100g/4oz	quark or skimmed milk cheese	½ cup
1 x 150g/5fl oz	carton low-fat natural yogurt	⅔ cup
225g/8oz	raspberries, fresh or frozen, puréed	2 cups
	intense artificial sweetener to taste	
2	kiwi fruit, peeled and sliced	2

1. Mix the soft cheese and yogurt together in a bowl. Add the raspberry purée and sweetener to taste.
2. Arrange the kiwi fruit in individual dishes or 1 large bowl, reserving 2 or 3 slices. Pour the raspberry mixture over the fruit and chill in a refrigerator before serving. Then decorate with the reserved kiwi fruit slices.

YOGURT GOOSEBERRY FOOL

CHO 10g/kcalories 160
Serves 6

Metric/Imperial		American
450g/1 lb	gooseberries, topped and tailed	1 lb
	intense artificial sweetener to taste	
1 x 150g/5fl oz	carton low-fat natural yogurt or diet gooseberry yogurt	⅔ cup
1–2 drops	green food colouring (optional)	1–2 drops

1. Put the gooseberries in a pan with a little water and cook them gently until the fruit is soft. Purée the gooseberries in a blender and press through a sieve to remove the seeds. Fold the yogurt into the fruit purée. Add 1–2 drops of green food colouring if using.
2. Divide the fool between 6 individual glass dessert bowls or wine goblets and chill until you are ready to serve.

Note to Cooks

Because each portion will have an insignificant amount of CHO, it does not have to be counted in the diet.

FRUIT AND YOGURT WHIPS

CHO 60g/kcalories 410
Serves 4

Metric/Imperial		American
1	banana, peeled and chopped	1
1 x 5ml sp/1 tsp	lemon juice	1 tsp
2	size 3 egg whites	2
1 x 15ml sp/ 1 tbs	intense artificial sweetener	1 tbs
2 x 150g/5fl oz	cartons low-fat natural yogurt	⅔ cup
25g/1oz	dried mixed fruit	2 tbs
25g/1oz	chopped hazelnuts	3 tbs

1. Mix the banana with the lemon juice in a bowl to prevent it browning.
2. Whisk the egg whites until they are stiff, then gently fold in the sweetener and yogurt using a metal spoon.
3. Fold in the dried fruit and nuts, reserving a little to decorate the whips.
4. Divide the mixture between 4 dishes and sprinkle each one with the reserved nuts. Serve immediately.

Note to Cooks

Try using a diet fruit-flavoured yogurt instead of the natural yogurt, say, apple and cinnamon, peach or apricot.

YOGURT SNOW WITH RASPBERRY SAUCE

CHO 20g/kcalories 160
Serves 3–4

Metric/Imperial		*American*
2 x 150g/5fl oz cartons	low-fat natural yogurt	1 cup
	intense artificial sweetener to taste	
1	egg white, beaten until stiff	1

Raspberry sauce

100g/4oz	raspberries	1 cup
1	lemon, juice of	1
	intense artificial sweetener to taste	
	a few mint leaves to decorate	

1. Drain the yogurt in a muslin-lined sieve for several hours (preferably overnight). Add the sweetener to the drained yogurt and fold in the beaten egg white. Spoon the Snow into ramekin dishes and chill for about an hour.
2. Meanwhile, purée the raspberries – reserving 3 or 4 to decorate – in a liquidizer for several minutes. Add the lemon juice and sweetener and purée again. Strain the sauce into a serving jug.
3. Decorate the Snow with the reserved raspberries and the mint leaves and serve the sauce in a jug for people to help themselves.

Note to Cooks

You can use a clean 'all-purpose cloth' if you don't happen to have any muslin.

APPLE DELIGHT

CHO 50g/kcalories 260
Serves 2

Metric/Imperial		*American*
2 x 150g/5fl oz	cartons low-fat natural yogurt	⅔ cup
2	eating apples, peeled, cored and grated	2
½	lemon, zest and juice of intense artificial sweetener to taste (optional)	½
2	walnut halves to decorate	2

1. Pour the yogurt into a bowl. Add the apple, lemon zest and juice and sweeten to taste.
2. Pour the Delight into 2 individual dishes and chill well before serving.
3. Top each dish with a walnut half and serve.

RASPBERRY MOUSSE

CHO 39.99g/kcalories 376
Serves 6–8

Metric/Imperial		*American*
1	sachet raspberry sugar-free jelly crystals	1
1 x 400g/14oz	can raspberries in natural juice	2 cups
2	size 3 egg whites	2
1 x 150ml/ 5fl oz	carton fromage frais	⅔ cup

1. Make the jelly up to 275ml/½ pint with boiling water.
2. Purée the raspberries and make up to 275ml/½ pint with water (sieve it to remove the pips if you prefer a smooth texture).
3. Add the raspberry mixture to the jelly and, once it has cooled, put it in the refrigerator until it has nearly set – until the jelly coats the back of a spoon (this usually takes about 1 hour).
4. Whisk the cream until it is thick and stir the fromage frais into the jelly mixture. Beat the egg whites until they are stiff and gently fold them into the jelly using a metal spoon.
5. Pour the mousse into a dish and leave it to set in the refrigerator.

Note to Cooks

An individual/single serving would have a negligible amount of CHO.

MARBLED APRICOTS

CHO 40g/kcalories 240
Serves 4-6

Metric/Imperial		*American*
450g/1 lb	fresh apricots, cut in half and the stones removed	2 cups
200g/7oz	fat-free fromage frais intense artificial sweetener to taste (optional)	1 cup

1. Stew the apricots in a little water until they are tender. Leave them to cool then purée them in a blender or food processor.
2. Pour the fromage frais into a 500ml/1 pint glass bowl, add the sweetener, if using, spoon in the apricot purée and blend only until a marble effect occurs – do not mix them together thoroughly.
3. Chill the mixture before serving.

PEARS CASSIS

CHO 80g/kcalories 320
Serves 4

Metric/Imperial		American
4	pears, peeled, cored and halved	4
275ml/½ pint	water	1⅓ cups
1 or	vanilla pod or	1 or
2–3 drops	vanilla essence	2–3 drops
275g/10oz	can blackcurrants in natural juice	1½ cups
	intense artificial sweetener to taste	
2 x 5ml sp/2 tsp	arrowroot	2 tsp

1. Put the pear halves in a pan with the water and vanilla. Cover the pan, bring to the boil, then simmer until the pears look almost transparent (this will take about 20–30 minutes).
2. Meanwhile, purée the blackcurrants.
3. When the pears are ready, drain them, reserving the cooking liquid, put them in a serving dish and keep them warm.
4. Make the blackcurrant purée up to 425ml/¾ pint with the reserved liquid from the pears, adding sweetener to taste, and heat it gently.
5. Mix the arrowroot with 2 tbs of the pear liquid and add it to the pan, stirring as you do so and until it thickens slightly, then pour it over the pears and serve.

CHEESECAKE

CHO 140g/kcalories 1600
Serves 6–8

Metric/Imperial		*American*
50g/2oz	low-fat spread	¼ cup
175g/6oz	wholemeal biscuits, crushed	1½ cups
1 sachet	gelatine	1 sachet
1	orange, finely grated rind and juice of	1
225g/8oz	skimmed milk cheese, quark or low-fat soft cheese	1 cup
1 x 150g/5fl oz	carton low-fat natural yogurt	⅔ cup
	liquid sweetener to taste	
2	size 3 eggs, separated	2
100g/4oz	fresh or frozen raspberries	1 cup

1. Melt the low-fat spread and mix it with the crushed biscuits. Press it down evenly in the bottom of an 18cm/7 inch spring release or a loose bottomed tin. Leave it to chill in the refrigerator for 30 minutes.
2. Meanwhile, dissolve gelatine in 3 tbs of hot water. Put the orange rind and juice and skimmed milk cheese or quark into a bowl. Add the yogurt, sweetener and egg yolks and mix them together well. Add the cooled gelatine and mix well. Whisk the egg whites until they are stiff and then lightly fold them into the yogurt mixture. Carefully pour the mixture into the tin, smooth the top and chill for several hours, preferably overnight.

3. Remove the cheesecake from the tin, leaving the base in place, and put it on a flat serving plate. Decorate the top with the raspberries.

Note to Cooks

You can freeze the cheesecake if you wish, but do so before putting the fruit on top and decorate it instead when you defrost it to use at a later date.

FRESH FRUIT JELLY

CHO 40g/kcalories 190
Serves 6-8

Metric/Imperial		American
1	packet sugar-free jelly crystals	1
1	red apple, cored and sliced	1
1	orange, peeled and segmented	1
20	grapes (10 black and 10 white)	20
	You can use any fresh fruit you like that is in season. Strawberries, bananas, tangerines and white grapes are all good alternatives.	

1. Make up the jelly crystals according to the directions on the packet.
2. Put the fruit into a bowl and pour the jelly over it. Leave it to cool then chill it until it has set in a refrigerator before serving.

PEACH ICE-CREAM

CHO 70g/kcalories 500
Serves 6–8

Metric/Imperial		*American*
1 x 425g/15oz	can peach slices in natural juice	2 cups
1 x 150g/5fl oz	carton low-fat natural yogurt	⅔ cup
1 x 170g/6–7oz	can evaporated milk, well chilled	¾ cup

1. Put the peaches and the juice into a blender or food processor and blend for 1–2 minutes.
2. Whisk the evaporated milk until it is thick and has doubled in volume. Whisk in the yogurt and gently fold the peach purée into the mixture.
3. Pour it into a freezer-proof container and freeze it until it has frozen around the edges (this takes about 1–2 hours). Beat the mixture breaking up the crystals and pour it back into the container or individual cartons and freeze it uncovered.
4. Put the ice-cream in a refrigerator for 10–15 minutes to soften a little before you serve it.

FRUIT FOOL

CHO 50g/kcalories 280
Serves 2

Metric/Imperial		American
175g/6oz	blackcurrants	1 cup
4 x 5ml sp/4 tsp	custard powder	4 tsp
150ml/¼ pint	skimmed milk	⅔ cup
1 x 150g/5fl oz	carton low-fat natural yogurt	⅔ cup
1 x 5ml sp/1 tsp	intense artificial sweetener	1 tsp

1. Cook the blackcurrants in approximately 2 tbs water until they are soft, then sieve or liquidize the fruit.
2. Make the custard by mixing the custard powder with 4 tsp of the milk, warming the rest of the milk, mixing in the custard powder mixture and stirring continuously until it thickens, then take it off the heat and leave it to cool.
3. When the custard has cooled, add the puréed fruit and yogurt to the custard and mix them together thoroughly. Sweeten the fool to taste and chill before serving.

GRAPE JELLY

CHO 30g/kcalories 190
Serves 6

Metric/Imperial		American
150ml/¼ pint	unsweetened white grape juice	⅔ cup
generous 3 x 15ml sp/ 3 tbs	lemon juice	generous 3 tbs
275ml/½ pint	water	1⅓ cups
15g/½ oz	gelatine, dissolved in 3 tbs cold water	1 tbs
	artificial sweetener to taste	
75g/3oz	small black or green grapes, halved and depipped	½ cup

1. Pour the grape and lemon juice and water into a dish. Add the dissolved gelatine, stirring, then chill the jelly until the mixture has the consistency of unbeaten egg white.
2. Stir in the grapes and chill until the jelly has set.

PEARS IN MULLED WINE

CHO 60g/kcalories 430
Serves 4

Metric/Imperial		American
4	ripe even-sized pears	4
275ml/½ pint	red wine	1⅓ cups
pinch	grated nutmeg	pinch
1 stick	cinnamon	1 stick
½	lemon, rind of	½
few drops	lemon juice	few drops
4	cloves	4
	intense artificial sweetener	
	to taste	

1. Peel the pears, leaving the stalks on. Slice a sliver off the bottom so that they will stand up.
2. Put all the ingredients, except the pears, into a saucepan and heat for 5 minutes. Pour everything into a small, deep-sided dish and stand the pears in it, basting them with the wine mixture.
3. Bake the pears at 350°F/180°C/gas mark 4 for 30 minutes, basting them occasionally.
4. Serve the pears immediately, with a little of the cooking juices dribbled over them.

SUMMER PUDDING

CHO 90g/kcalories 610
Serves 6

Metric/Imperial		American
675g/1½–2 lb	mixed soft fruits, such as	1½–2 lb
	blackcurrants, redcurrants,	
	raspberries and blackberries	
	intense artificial sweetener	
	to taste	
about 6	slices of stale white bread,	about 6
	crusts removed	

1. Put the soft fruits in a saucepan and cook them gently for 5 minutes or until the juices run and the fruits soften and sweeten to taste.
2. Meanwhile, line the bottom and sides of a 825ml/1½ pint pudding basin with the bread, ensuring that there are no gaps between the slices and reserving 1½ slices for the top.
3. Put the fruit and all but 2 x 15ml sp/2 tbs of the juice into the bread-lined basin, cover with the reserved bread. Put a plate over the top and weigh it down with weights or a heavy tin. Chill the pudding overnight.
4. To unmould the pudding, hold the serving plate, inverted, over the top of the basin and turn the pudding over. Pour the reserved fruit juice over the pudding just before serving.

10

Home Baking

HOME-BAKED bread and teatime treats are pleasures that shouldn't be a thing of the past. You can still enjoy them if you like to treat yourself occasionally. They needn't take long to make either and beat bought versions hands down.

The recipes for traditional favourites here have been modified so that high-fibre, low-fat and low-sugar ingredients are used. Try some with your afternoon tea today!

WHOLEMEAL BREAD

CHO 580g/kcalories 2990
Makes 3 450g/1 lb loaves

Metric/Imperial		*American*
900g/2 lb	wholemeal flour	8 cups
1 x 15ml sp/ 1 tbs	salt	1 tbs
50g/2oz	low-fat spread	¼ cup
1 x 15ml sp/ 1 tbs	easy-blend dried yeast	1 tbs
1 x 15ml sp/ 1 tbs	malt extract	1 tbs
550ml/1 pint	tepid water	2½ cups

1. Combine the flour, salt and yeast, then rub in the low-fat spread. Dissolve the yeast and the malt in the water and gradually add it to the flour, mixing it in well. Knead it to a soft dough, then turn it out onto a floured board and knead for 10–15 minutes until it is smooth and elastic.

2. Divide the mixture into 3 and put each in a lightly oiled 450g/1 lb loaf tin. Put them in a warm place to prove (double in size).

3. Bake them at 400°F/200°C/gas mark 6 for 10 minutes then reduce the temperature to 350°F/180°C/gas mark 4 for 25–35 minutes. You can tell that they are done if when you turn them out they sound hollow when you rap the bottoms. Turn them out of the tins and leave them to cool on a wire rack.

Note to Cooks

These loaves freeze well wrapped in foil once they have cooled.

VICTORIA SANDWICH

CHO 120g/kcalories 1060
Serves 8

Metric/Imperial		American
100g/4oz	low-fat spread	½ cup
50g/2oz	caster sugar	⅓ cup
2	size 3 eggs, lightly beaten	2
1 x 15ml sp/ 1 tbs	hot water	1 tbs
100g/4oz	self-raising wholemeal flour	1 cup
pinch	baking powder	pinch

1. Cream the low-fat spread and sugar together until the mixture is light and creamy. Beat in the eggs and water. Sieve the flour and baking powder into another bowl, then gradually add it to the creamed mixture, folding it in so that they are thoroughly mixed together.

2. Divide the mixture between 2 15cm/6 inch, lightly greased sandwich tins and bake at 350°F/180°C/gas mark 4 for 20–25 minutes until they have risen well, spring back when touched and are golden brown. Turn them out onto a wire tray to cool.

3. You can then fill the cake with pure fruit spread and whipped cream and sprinkle a little powdered intense sweetener over the top or fill it with pure fruit spread and some of the Butter Icing recipe on page 240. A pretty finishing touch is to lay a paper doily on top of the filled cake and sift a little powdered sweetener over it. When you lift the doily, there will be a lacy pattern.

Note to Cooks

If you use jam in the cake remember to add the CHO and calories. 1 oz pure fruit spread contains approx. 10g CHO, 35 cals. If using whipped cream a 142ml/5fl oz carton contains 510 calories.

FAIRY CAKES

CHO 90g/kcalories 660
Makes 10

Metric/Imperial		*American*
50g/2oz	low-fat spread	¼ cup
25g/1oz	caster sugar	2 tbs
1	size 3 egg, beaten	1
50g/2oz	self-raising wholemeal flour	½ cup
50g/2oz	raisins	⅓ cup
1 x 15ml sp/ 1 tbs	boiling water, if needed	1 tbs

1. Cream the low-fat spread and sugar together until the mixture pales in colour. Add half the beaten egg and 1 x 5ml sp/1 tsp of the flour and beat well. Add the remaining egg and 1 x 5ml sp/1 tsp of the flour and beat well. Add the remaining flour gradually and the raisins, folding them in gently using a metal spoon. The mixture should now be of a dropping consistency (if it is not, add the 1 x 15ml sp/1 tbs of boiling water).
2. Spoon equal amounts of the mixture into 10 paper cases in a patty tin and bake on the middle shelf of the oven for 10–15 minutes at 350°F/180°C/gas mark 4 until the Fairy Cakes have risen well, are golden brown and firm to the touch.

BUTTERFLY CAKES

CHO 120g/kcalories 1160
Makes 12–15

Metric/Imperial		*American*
1	Victoria Sandwich recipe (see page 220) a little granular intense artificial sweetener Butter Icing recipe (see page 240) flavoured with 1–2 drops vanilla essence	1

1. Prepare the Victoria Sandwich recipe as given on page 220 and divide the mixture between 12–15 paper cases in patty tins. Bake them in a 350°F/180°C/gas mark 4 oven for 12–15 minutes until the Cakes have risen and are golden brown. Remove them from the tin and leave them to cool on a wire rack.

2. Meanwhile, prepare the Butter Icing as given on page 240.

3. When the Cakes have cooled, cut a slice from the top of each bun and put a tsp of the Butter Icing over the cut cake. Cut the removed slices in half and place them on the cakes, angling them into the Butter Icing to form 'wings'. Dust the Cakes with granular intense artificial sweetener. The cakes are tastiest when they are fresh.

BANANA AND WALNUT SLICES

CHO 160g/kcalories 1580
Makes 16

Metric/Imperial		American
100g/4oz	low-fat spread	½ cup
50g/2oz	sugar	⅓ cup
2	size 3 eggs	2
100g/4oz	wholemeal self-raising flour	1 cup
1 x 5ml sp/1 tsp	baking powder	1 tsp
2 small	bananas, mashed	2 small
75g/3oz	walnuts, chopped	⅔ cup

1. Preheat the oven to 375°F/190°C/gas mark 5.
2. Cream the low-fat spread and the sugar together until the mixture is light and fluffy. Beat in the eggs, one at a time, adding a tbs of the flour with the second egg. Fold in the remaining flour and the baking powder together with the bananas.
3. Spread the mixture evenly in a lined and greased 15 by 25cm/6 by 10 inch shallow tin and sprinkle the walnuts over the top. Bake in the preheated oven for 20–25 minutes.
4. When the mixture has cooked, leave it in the tin but cut it into 16 equal pieces. Leave the tin on a wire rack to cool, then turn the slices out and store them in an airtight container.

TEA BREAD

CHO 210g/kcalories 1680
Makes 1 450g/1 lb loaf

Metric/Imperial		American
100g/4oz	low-fat spread	½ cup
50g/2oz	caster sugar	⅛ cup
1	size 3 egg, beaten	1
2 small	bananas, mashed	2 small
1 x 150g/5fl oz	carton low-fat natural yogurt	⅔ cup
50g/2oz	white self-raising flour	½ cup
100g/4oz	wholemeal self-raising flour	1 cup
50g/2oz	walnuts, chopped	½ cup
25g/1oz	sultanas	2 tbs

1. Cream the low-fat spread and sugar until the mixture is light and fluffy. Add the egg and beat it in well. Stir in the bananas and yogurt. Gently fold in the flour, walnuts and sultanas.

2. Spoon the mixture into a lightly greased 450g/1 lb loaf tin and bake at 375°F/190°C/gas mark 5 for approximately 1 hour or until it is cooked (check it by inserting a clean skewer into the centre and leaving it there for a couple of seconds – if it comes out clean, the Tea Bread is done).

Home Baking

RHUBARB AND RAISIN CAKE

CHO 210g/kcalories 1260
Makes 12 portions

Metric/Imperial		*American*
225g/8oz	rhubarb, chopped	½ lb
50g/2oz	low-fat spread	¼ cup
225g/8oz	self-raising wholemeal flour	2 cups
1 x 5ml sp/1 tsp	baking powder	1 tsp
100g/4oz	raisins	⅔ cup
1	size 3 egg, beaten	1
4 x 15ml sp/ 4 tbs	skimmed milk	4 tbs

1. Cook the rhubarb in a little water for 5–10 minutes.
2. Rub the low-fat spread into the flour and baking powder, which you have sieved together into a bowl. Add the rhubarb and raisins and mix them in. Add the egg and milk and mix them in well.
3. Pour the mixture into a lightly oiled 18cm/7 inch cake tin and bake at 375°F/190°C/gas mark 5 for 1 hour. Turn the cake out and leave it to cool on a wire rack.

Note to Cooks

This cake freezes well. Just wrap it in foil once it has cooled.

CELEBRATION CAKE

CHO 320g/kcalories 2300
Makes 24 portions

Metric/Imperial		*American*
25g/1oz	sugar	2 tbs
75g/3oz	sultanas	½ cup
75g/3oz	currants	½ cup
75g/3oz	raisins	½ cup
300ml/½ pint	Guinness	1⅓ cups
50g/2oz	low-fat spread	¼ cup
225g/8oz	100 per cent wholemeal flour	2 cups
1 x 2.5ml sp/ ½ tsp	baking powder	½ tsp
1 x 5ml sp/1 tsp	mixed spice	1 tsp
75g/3oz	walnuts, chopped	⅔ cup
3	size 3 eggs, beaten	3

1. Put the sugar, fruit and Guinness in a pan, bring it to the boil, then leave it to simmer for 20 minutes. Add the low-fat spread and leave it to cool. Add the beaten egg to the mixture. Sieve the flour and baking powder together into a bowl, then stir it into the pan.
2. Pour the mixture into a well-oiled 18cm/7 inch square tin and bake at 350°F/180°C/gas mark 4 for 1–1½ hours. Leave it to cool in the tin on a wire rack.
3. To test whether the Cake is cooked, insert a clean skewer into the centre and leave it there for 2 seconds. If the skewer if clean when you pull it out, the cake is done.

Home Baking

Note to Cooks

This cake freezes well wrapped in foil.

DATE AND WALNUT LOAF

CHO 370g/kcalories 2290
Makes 1 900g/2 lb loaf

Metric/Imperial		American
225g/8oz	stoned dates, chopped	1⅓ cups
1 x 2.5ml sp/ ½ tsp	bicarbonate of soda	½ tsp
1 x 2.5ml sp/ ½ tsp	salt	½ tsp
150ml/¼ pint	boiling water	⅔ cup
100g/4oz	low-fat spread	½ cup
75g/3oz	brown sugar	½ cup
1	size 3 egg, beaten	1
225g/8oz	wholemeal self-raising flour	2 cups
50g/2oz	walnuts, chopped	½ cup

1. Put the dates, bicarbonate of soda and salt in a basin, pour the boiling water over them and put to one side.

2. Meanwhile, cream the low-fat spread and sugar and beat in the egg. Stir in flour, nuts and date mixture and stir until all the ingredients are combined. Pour the mixture into a lightly greased 900g/2 lb loaf tin and bake at 350°F/180°C/gas mark 4 for 1–1½ hours. To test whether the Loaf is done, poke a clean skewer into the centre of it, leave it there for 2 seconds, then if it comes out clean, it is done.

3. Then turn it out onto a wire rack and leave it to cool. When it has cooled, store in an airtight container.

PRUNE AND NUT CAKE

CHO 190g/kcalories 1310
Makes 12 portions

Metric/Imperial		*American*
225g/8oz	self-raising wholemeal flour	2 cups
pinch	salt	pinch
1 x 5ml sp/1 tsp	grated nutmeg	1 tsp
1 small	orange, grated zest of	1 small
25g/1oz	low-fat spread	2 tbs
50g/2oz	walnuts, chopped	½ cup
75g/3oz	stoneless prunes, chopped	½ cup
1	size 3 egg, beaten	1
100ml/3fl oz	skimmed milk	⅓ cup
3 x 15ml sp/ 3 tbs	juice from the orange	3 tbs

1. Sieve the flour, salt and spices into a bowl and add the orange zest. Mix in the low-fat spread using a fork. Stir in the walnuts and prunes and beat in the egg, milk and orange juice until everything is well mixed.
2. Turn the mixture into a greased 15cm/6 inch round cake tin and bake at 375°F/190°C/gas mark 5 for 40–45 minutes or until the Cake is well risen and golden brown and a skewer pierced through the centre of the cake comes out clean.
3. Allow it to cool before serving.

Note to Cooks

Serve this with Curd Cheese Topping (see page 239) for a special occasion.

ROCK CAKES

CHO 230g/kcalories 1460
Makes 14

Metric/Imperial		American
100g/4oz	self-raising wholemeal flour	1 cup
100g/4oz	self-raising white flour	1 cup
100g/4oz	low-fat spread	½ cup
50g/2oz	granulated sugar	⅓ cup
50g/2oz	currants	⅓ cup
1	size 3 egg, beaten	1
75ml/⅛ pint	skimmed milk	¼ cup

1. Sieve the flours into a mixing bowl. Rub the low-fat spread into the flours until the mixture resembles fine breadcrumbs. Then stir in the sugar and currants.
2. Make a well in the centre and pour the beaten egg and milk into it. Mix all the ingredients together, stirring round in the well, gradually incorporating all the dry ingredients.
3. Make 14 even-sized mounds of the mixture on a greased baking sheet and bake at 400°F/200°C/gas mark 6 for 10–15 minutes.
4. Leave the Rock Cakes to cool on a wire rack before serving them.

MAIDS OF HONOUR

CHO 200g/kcalories 1570
Makes 15–16

Metric/Imperial		*American*
Pastry		
100g/4oz	wholemeal flour	1 cup
50g/2oz	white flour	½ cup
pinch	salt	pinch
50g/2oz	low-fat spread	¼ cup
25g/1oz	white polyunsaturated vegetable fat	2 tbs
	a little cold water to mix	

Filling		
8 x 5ml sp/8 tsp	pure fruit spread	8 tsp
50g/2oz	low-fat spread	¼ cup
25g/1oz	caster sugar	2 tbs
1	size 3 egg, beaten	1
50g/2oz	self-raising wholemeal flour	½ cup

1. Make the pastry by sieving the flours and salt into a bowl and rubbing the fats into the flour and stirring a little cold water into the mixture to bind it together.
2. Refrigerate the pastry for 30 minutes, then roll it out and, using a 7cm/3 inch round pastry cutter, cut out 15–16 shapes and put them in lightly greased patty tins. Put a half teaspoonful of the pure fruit spread in the bottom of each.

3. Cream the low-fat spread and sugar until the mixture is creamy, then fold in the beaten egg and flour. Put a small spoonful of the mixture in each case and bake them at 400°F/200°C/gas mark 6 for 15–20 minutes.

4. Leave them to cool on a wire rack.

MADELEINES

CHO 150g/kcalories 1760
Makes 10

Metric/Imperial		American
1	Victoria Sandwich recipe (see page 220)	1
75g/3oz	reduced-sugar raspberry jam, warmed	¼ cup
100g/4oz	desiccated coconut	1⅓ cups
5	glacé cherries, halved	5
	angelica leaves to decorate	

1. Make the Victoria Sandwich mixture as given on page 220.
2. Spoon the mixture into 10 lightly greased dariole moulds so that they are ⅔ full and bake at 350°F/ 180°C/gas mark 4 for approximately 15 minutes or until the mixture has risen and turned golden brown.
3. Loosen the Madeleines round the edges with a knife and turn them out onto a cooling rack. When they are cool, thinly spread the jam over them and roll them in the coconut until they are coated in it. Put a glacé cherry on top of each cake and angelica leaves each side of it.

JAM TARTS

CHO 130g/kcalories 890
Makes 18–20

Metric/Imperial		*American*
75g/3oz	wholemeal flour	¾ cup
25g/1oz	plain flour	¼ cup
25g/1oz	low-fat spread	2 tbs
25g/1oz	white polyunsaturated vegetable fat	2 tbs
2 x 15ml sp/ 2 tbs	cold water	2 tbs
1 x 5ml sp/1 tsp	polyunsaturated oil	1 tsp
6–6½ x 15ml sp/ 6–6½ tbs	reduced-sugar jam	6–6½ tbs

1. Make the pastry by sieving the flours together into a bowl, rubbing the fats into the flours until the mixture resembles fine breadcrumbs, then adding the water and oil and working the mixture into a dough.
2. Chill the pastry for 30 minutes before rolling it out on a lightly floured surface. Using a 5cm/2 inch pastry cutter, cut out 18–20 rounds, gathering the scraps together and rolling it out again as necessary to use up as much of the pastry as possible.
3. Put the pastry circles in lightly greased patty tins and put a teaspoonful of jam into each. Bake for 15–20 minutes at 400°F/200°C/gas mark 6. Cool them on a wire rack.

CINNAMON SCONE

CHO 170g/kcalories 1100
Serves 8–10

Metric/Imperial		American
225g/8oz	self-raising wholemeal flour	2 cups
pinch	salt	pinch
2 x 5ml sp/2 tsp	baking powder	2 tsp
3 x 5ml sp/3 tsp	cinnamon	3 tsp
50g/2oz	low-fat spread	¼ cup
1 x 15ml sp/ 1 tbs	caster sugar	1 tbs
1	size 3 egg, lightly beaten	1
about 150ml/¼ pint	skimmed milk	⅔ cup
1 x 5ml sp/1 tsp	intense artificial sweetener	1 tsp

1. Sieve the flour, salt, baking powder and 2 tsp of the cinnamon into a bowl and rub in the low-fat spread until the mixture resembles fine breadcrumbs.
2. Stir in the sugar then gradually pour in the egg and milk and stir the mixture until it forms a soft dough. Turn it onto a floured surface, knead it gently until it is smooth, then roll the dough out into a round approximately 18cm/7 inch in diameter and 2.5cm/1 inch thick.
3. Put the Scone on a lightly greased baking sheet and score it into 8 portions. Brush the surface with milk and sprinkle the remaining cinnamon over the top. Bake it at 425°F/220°C/gas mark 7 for 15–20 minutes

Home Baking

until the scone has risen and is firm to the touch.

4. Sprinkle the intense artificial sweetener over the scone once it comes out of the oven.

RICH SCONES

CHO 210g/kcalories 1230
Makes 12–14

Metric/Imperial		*American*
225g/8oz	self-raising wholemeal flour	2 cups
1 x 2.5ml sp/ ½ tsp	salt	½ tsp
50g/2oz	low-fat spread	¼ cup
25g/1oz	sugar	2 tbs
50g/2oz	sultanas	⅓ cup
1	size 3 egg, beaten with sufficient skimmed milk to make it up to 150ml/¼ pint/ ⅔ cup	1

1. Sieve the flour and salt together into a bowl and rub the low-fat spread into them. Stir in the sugar and sultanas. Add the egg and milk, reserving enough to glaze the tops later.
2. Knead the resulting dough lightly on a floured surface and roll it out to an even 2.5cm/1 inch thickness. Using a 5cm/2 inch pastry cutter, cut out as many rounds as you can, gathering together the scraps and rolling it out again to use as much of the dough as you can.
3. Put them on a lightly greased baking sheet and brush the tops with the reserved liquid. Bake them in a hot oven at 425°F/220°C/gas mark 7 for approximately 10 minutes, then cool them on a wire rack.

Home Baking

CURD CHEESE TOPPING

CHO neg/kcalories 130
Sufficient for a 18cm/7 inch cake

Metric/Imperial		American
75g/3oz	curd cheese	⅓ cup
	liquid intense artificial	
	sweetener to taste	
	flavouring and/or	
	colouring (optional)	

1. Beat the curd cheese until it is smooth and fairly soft.
2. Add the sweetener to taste and colouring or flavouring if liked.

Note to Cooks

Use the topping just to sandwich cakes together or to decorate the top as well.

BUTTER ICING

CHO neg/kcalories 100
Sufficient for 6 small cakes

Metric/Imperial		*American*
2 x 15ml sp/ 2 tbs	powdered intense artificial sweetener	2 tbs
25g/1oz	low-fat spread	2 tbs

1. Beat the ingredients together to form a smooth paste, shortly before you intend using it.

Note to Cooks

This versatile icing can be flavoured in a variety of ways depending on what you like and the cake you are decorating. Try a few drops of vanilla essence or a tablespoon of cocoa powder or a teaspoon of coffee essence.

11

Festive Occasions

FESTIVE TIMES need not be a time of denial. Try these tasty adaptations of traditional favourites and you'll be doing yourself good without you or your guests even noticing. You can feel confident that at Christmas, especially, a time when good food is at the centre of all the festivities, you, your family and friends can all enjoy a feast of *good* things – in all senses of the word.

BROCCOLI AND MUSHROOM FLAN

CHO 110g/kcalories 1710
Serves 6–8

Metric/Imperial		*American*
Pastry		
100g/4oz	wholemeal flour	1 cup
50g/2oz	plain flour	½ cup
pinch	salt	pinch
50g/2oz	low-fat spread	¼ cup
25g/1oz	white polyunsaturated vegetable fat	2 tbs
	a little cold water to bind	

Filling		
225g/8oz	broccoli cut into small florets	2 cups
100g/4oz	mushrooms, sliced	1½ cups
1	clove garlic, crushed	
100g/4oz	reduced-fat cheddar cheese, grated	1 cup
2	size 3 eggs, lightly beaten	2
1 x 150g/5fl oz	carton single cream	⅔ cup
	salt and freshly ground black pepper	

1. Make the pastry first. Sieve the flours and salt into a bowl. Rub the fats into the flours until the mixture resembles fine breadcrumbs, then mix in a little cold

water to work it into a dough. Chill the pastry for 30 minutes before rolling it out to line a 26cm/10 inch flan tin or dish. Bake the pastry case blind for 10 minutes at 350°F/180°C/gas mark 4.

2. Meanwhile, steam or boil the broccoli florets until they have cooked through but are still a little crisp. Arrange them evenly over the bottom of the flan case, then sprinkle in the mushrooms and spread the garlic over the vegetables. Cover them with the cheese. Beat the eggs with the cream and season to taste with salt and freshly ground black pepper. Pour this mixture into the flan case and bake it at 325°F/170°C/gas mark 3 for approximately 45 minutes or until the egg and cream mixture has set.

PRAWN AND RICE RING

CHO 150g/kcalories 1440
Serves 10

Metric/Imperial		*American*
Ring		
175g/6oz	brown rice, cooked	1 cup
275g/10oz	frozen mixed vegetables, blanched	2½ cups
Dressing		
4 x 15ml sp/ 4 tbs	olive oil	4 tbs
2 x 15ml sp/ 2tbs	wine vinegar	2 tbs
pinch	dry mustard salt and freshly ground black pepper	pinch
Filling		
2 x 15ml sp/ 2 tbs	low-calorie mayonnaise	2 tbs
1 x 15ml sp/ 1 tbs	tomato ketchup	1 tbs
few drops	Worcestershire sauce	few drops
225g/8oz	prawns lemon twist, to garnish	2 cups

1. Add the vegetables to the rice. Then combine all the dressing ingredients in a screw-top jar and shake it well. Stir just enough of the dressing into the rice mixture to make it glisten, then spoon into a ring mould and press down into it well. Chill it well.

2. Meanwhile, make the filling. Combine the mayonnaise, ketchup, Worcestershire sauce and prawns and stir them all together well. Carefully turn the rice ring out onto a serving dish and fill the centre with the prawn mixture. Garnish it with a twist of lemon and serve.

SALMON QUICHE

CHO 910g/kcalories 1560
Serves 6

Metric/Imperial		American
Pastry		
100g/4oz	wholemeal flour	1 cup
50g/2oz	plain flour	½ cup
pinch	salt	pinch
50g/2oz	low-fat spread	¼ cup
25g/1oz	white polyunsaturated fat	2 tbs
	a little cold water to mix	
Filling		
1 x 200g/7oz	can pink salmon, drained and flaked	1 cup
100g/4oz	cottage cheese, drained	½ cup
2	size 3 eggs, lightly beaten	2
2 x 15ml sp/ 2 tbs	skimmed milk	2 tbs
	freshly ground black pepper	
1	tomato, sliced	

1. Make the pastry. Sieve the flours and salt into a bowl. Rub in the fats until the mixture resembles fine breadcrumbs. Stir in enough water to bind the mixture into a soft dough.
2. Chill the pastry for 30 minutes before rolling it out to line a 26cm/10 inch flan tin or dish. Bake the pastry

case blind for 10 minutes at 400°F/200°C/gas mark 6. When it has cooked, spoon the flaked salmon evenly over the bottom.

3. Now make the filling. Liquidize or blend the cottage cheese, eggs, and milk until the mixture becomes smooth. Season it with freshly ground black pepper and pour it over the salmon. Arrange the tomato slices on top and bake at 400°F/200°C/gas mark 6 for 30–35 minutes or until the cheese, egg and milk mixture has set.

MUSHROOM AND ONION STUFFING

CHO 40g/kcalories 490

Metric/Imperial		*American*
25g/1oz	low-fat spread	2 tbs
1 x 15ml sp/ 1 tbs	corn or sunflower oil	1 tbs
100g/4oz	mushrooms, sliced	1½ cups
1	onion, peeled and chopped	1
100g/4oz	wholemeal breadcrumbs	2 cups
1 x 15ml sp/ 1 tbs	fresh parsley, chopped	1 tbs
	salt and freshly ground black pepper	
	a little skimmed milk to bind, if necessary	

1. Melt the low-fat spread and oil in a pan and lightly fry the mushrooms and onion until they have softened.
2. Transfer the mixture to a mixing bowl and stir in the remaining ingredients, seasoning with salt and freshly ground black pepper to taste. Make sure the ingredients are well combined. Stir in a little milk to bind the mixture if necessary.
3. Use to stuff a chicken or turkey.

BREAD SAUCE

CHO 60g/kcalories 390
Makes approx 275ml/½ pint

Metric/Imperial		American
1	onion, peeled and quartered	1
425ml/¾ pint	skimmed milk	2 cups
6	black peppercorns	6
1	bay leaf	1
1	blade mace	1
3	cloves	3
100g/4oz	fresh wholemeal breadcrumbs	2 cups
pinch	salt	pinch

1. Put the onion, milk, herbs and spices in a saucepan and bring to the boil.
2. Remove the pan from the heat, cover it tightly and leave it to infuse for 15–20 minutes.
3. Strain out the herbs and spices and return the milk to the pan once you have rinsed it out. Add the breadcrumbs and salt to taste.
4. Simmer the sauce gently to reheat the milk, stirring occasionally. Adjust the seasoning to taste just before serving.

CHRISTMAS CAKE

CHO 500g/kcalories 4360
Makes 36 portions

Metric/Imperial		American
175g/6oz	sultanas	1 cup
175g/6oz	raisins	1 cup
100g/4oz	currants	⅔ cup
50g/2oz	glacé cherries, chopped	⅓ cup
275ml/½ pint	cold tea	1⅓ cups
200g/7oz	polyunsaturated margarine	14 tbs
50g/2oz	ground almonds	½ cup
275g/10oz	wholemeal flour	2½ cups
2 x 5ml sp/2 tsp	baking powder	2 tsp
2 x 5ml sp/2 tsp	mixed spice	2 tsp
3	size 3 eggs, beaten	3
1	lemon, grated rind of	1
50g/2oz	blanched almonds, chopped	½ cup

1. Put all the dried fruit into a bowl, cover it with the cold tea and leave the fruit to plump up overnight.
2. Cream the margarine and ground almonds until the mixture has lightened in colour. Sieve the flour, baking powder and mixed spice into a bowl and then gradually add the eggs and half the flour mixture to the creamed mixture. Fold in the lemon rind and chopped nuts. Carefully fold the remaining flour into the fruit mixture to make a soft dropping consistency. Pour the mixture into a greased and lined 20cm/8 inch cake tin.

3. Bake the cake at 325°F/170°C/gas mark 3 for 1 hour then reduce the heat to 275°F/140°C/gas mark 1 for a further 1–1¼ hours. Cover the top of the cake with greaseproof paper if it is browning too quickly.

4. To test whether the cake is done, push a clean skewer into the centre, leave it there for 2 seconds and if it comes out clean, the cake is cooked. Leave the cake to cool in its tin before turning it out. To store the cake, wrap it in foil or leave it 1 day to mature and then freeze it.

MARZIPAN

CHO 80g/kcalories 950

Metric/Imperial		American
100g/4oz	ground almonds	⅔ cup
50g/2oz	caster sugar	⅓ cup
25g/1oz	white flour	¼ cup
1	size 3 egg	1

1. Beat all the ingredients together to form a smooth paste. You can do this by hand or use a food processor.
2. Divide the mixture into two and wrap it in cling film and store it in a cool place if you are not using it straight away.

Note to Cooks

This recipe makes enough marzipan to cover the top and sides of an 18cm/7 inch cake.

DUNDEE CAKE

CHO 340g/kcalories 2520
Makes 16 portions

Metric/Imperial		American
175g/6oz	low-fat spread	¾ cup
50g/2oz	caster sugar	⅓ cup
225g/8oz	fine wholemeal self-raising flour	2 cups
pinch	salt	pinch
1 x 5ml sp/1 tsp	mixed spice	1 tsp
3	size 3 eggs, beaten	3
1 x 15ml sp/ 1 tbs	skimmed milk	1 tbs
200g/7oz	mixed fruit	1¼ cups
25g/1oz	split almonds for decoration	¼ cup

1. Cream the low-fat spread and sugar until the mixture is light and fluffy. Mix the flour together with the salt and mixed spice. Add the eggs to the creamed mixture, one at a time, with a little of the flour mixture, stirring and then beating the mixture thoroughly after each addition. Stir in the milk and beat again. Add the fruit and the rest of the flour mixture, folding them in lightly.
2. Spoon the mixture into a greased and lined 18cm/7 inch round cake tin. Arrange the split almonds on top in the traditional pattern of concentric circles and bake for 1 hour at 350°F/180°C/gas mark 4 and for a further 1–1¼ hours at 300°F/150°C/gas mark 2.

3. To check whether it is done, poke a clean skewer into the centre of the cake, leave it there for 2 seconds and, if when you remove it the skewer is clean, your cake is done. Then leave it to cool in the tin on a cooling rack before turning it out.

MINCE PIES

CHO 170g/kcalories 1150
Makes 12–16

Metric/Imperial		*American*
Pastry		
100g/4oz	wholemeal flour	1 cup
50g/2oz	plain flour	½ cup
50g/2oz	low-fat spread	¼ cup
25g/1oz	white polyunsaturated vegetable fat	2 tbs
	a little cold water to bind	

Filling

4–4½ x 15ml sp/ mincemeat 4–4½ tbs		4–4½ tbs
	a little milk to glaze	
	a little powdered intense artificial sweetener	

1. Make the pastry by sieving the flours together, rubbing in the fats until the mixture resembles breadcrumbs, then stir in a little water to make a soft dough.
2. Leave the pastry to chill in the refrigerator for 30 minutes, then roll it out on a lightly floured surface. Using a 5cm/2 inch pastry cutter and a small star cutter, cut out an equal number of bases and stars. Gather the scraps together and roll it out again to use the maximum amount of pastry.

3. Put the pastry circles in lightly greased patty tins and put 1 x 5ml sp/1 tsp of the mincemeat into each. Place a star on top of the mincemeat.
4. Bake the Mince Pies at 400°F/200°C/gas mark 6. When they are cooked, brush the stars with the milk and sprinkle a little of the sweetener over the top.

CHRISTMAS PUDDING

CHO 460g/kcalories 2920
Makes 2 x 550ml/1 pint puddings; each pudding serves 12

Metric/Imperial		*American*
200g/7oz	wholemeal breadcrumbs	4 cups
50g/2oz	dark brown sugar	1/3 cup
100g/4oz	vegetable suet	1/2 cup
pinch	salt	pinch
1 x 5ml sp/1 tsp	mixed spice	1 tsp
175g/6oz	sultanas	1 cup
175g/6oz	raisins	1 cup
100g/4oz	currants	2/3 cup
25g/1oz	blanched almonds, chopped	3 tbs
1 medium	cooking apple, peeled, cored and grated	1 medium
1	lemon, grated rind and juice of	1
1	size 3 egg, beaten	1
150ml/¼ pint	Guinness	2/3 cup
approx.	skimmed milk, if necessary	approx.
5 x 15ml sp/ 5 tbs		5 tbs

1. Mix the dry ingredients with the lemon juice, egg and Guinness, mixing them together well. Add a little milk if the mixture is too stiff.
2. Pour the mixture into 2 550ml/1 pint pudding basins that have been lightly oiled. Cover them lightly with greaseproof paper and foil and steam for 2–3 hours or

pressure cook at high pressure for 1–2 hours (consult the manufacturer's guide for your particular model).

3. Cover the puddings with fresh greaseproof paper and foil to store them. When you want to reheat them steam for 2 hours.

STUFFED DATES

CHO 170g/kcalories 1050
Makes 16

Metric/Imperial		American
16	fresh dates	16
½	Marzipan recipe (see page 252)	½
16	petit four cases	16

1. Remove the stones from the dates, then fill each cavity with a little marzipan and put the date in a petit four case.

EASTER BISCUITS

CHO 190g/kcalories 1290
Makes 28–30

Metric/Imperial		*American*
100g/4oz	low-fat spread	⅓ cup
50g/2oz	sugar	⅓ cup
1	size 3 egg, separated and white beaten	1
100g/4oz	wholemeal flour	1 cup
50g/2oz	rice flour	¼ cup
1 x 5ml sp/1 tsp	mixed spice	1 tsp
50g/2oz	currants	⅓ cup
1 x 15ml sp/ 1 tbs	skimmed milk, if necessary	1 tbs

1. Cream the low-fat spread and sugar together until the mixture is pale and creamy. Beat in the egg yolk then fold in the flours and mixed spice. Stir in the currants. If the dough is too stiff, mix in the milk to achieve a soft, pliable dough.
2. Knead the dough until it is smooth, then roll it out on a lightly floured surface. Cut out 28–30 rounds using a 5cm/2 inch pastry cutter. Gather the scraps together and roll it out again to waste as little dough as you can.
3. Place the biscuits on a lightly greased baking sheet and bake them in the centre of the oven at 400°F/ 200°C/gas mark 6 for about 10 minutes.

4. Brush the tops with the beaten egg white and return them to the oven to bake for about another 5 minutes. Cool them on a wire rack. When they have cooled, store them in an airtight container.

HOT FRUITY PUNCH

CHO 60g/kcalories 1890
Serves 12

Metric/Imperial		*American*
3	apples, cut into 8 pieces	3
3	oranges, cut into 8 pieces	3
12	whole cloves	12
2	cinnamon sticks	2
2	bottles red wine	2
550ml/1 pint	dry sherry	2½ cups
550ml/1 pint	unsweetened apple juice	2½ cups
1	orange, thinly sliced to decorate	

1. Put the apple and orange pieces into a large pan with the cloves and cinnamon sticks and pour the red wine over them. Bring it to the boil and simmer, covered, for 10 minutes.
2. Remove the pan from the heat and let it stand for 10 minutes for the flavours to infuse.
3. Strain the wine and discard the spices, return the wine to the pan, pour in the apple juice and sherry and heat until the liquid starts to bubble at the edges of the pan.
4. Pour the wine into a warm serving bowl and float the orange slices on top. Serve immediately.

12

Ideas for Children

CHILDREN LOVE to try different food, snacks, treats and drinks as much as adults do. As the majority of children are active and growing, it is even more important to provide them with healthy, nourishing meals. Quick food doesn't have to be junk food: why not try the American-style Hamburgers with the Bean Salad and homemade real Strawberry Milkshake?

You can make sure that there are plenty of protein foods in their diet by including meat, poultry, fish, dairy products, eggs and pulses. Vary what you give them and then you can be sure that they are eating a balanced diet and are less likely to become faddy eaters.

SANDWICH FILLINGS

Makes 1 round

Metric/Imperial		American
Skimmed Milk Cheese & Peanut Butter		
CHO 30g/kcalories 400		
1 x 15ml sp/ 1 tbs	crunchy peanut butter	1 tbs
2 x 15ml sp/ 2 tbs	skimmed milk cheese or low-fat soft cheese salt and freshly ground black pepper	2 tbs
2 slices	wholemeal bread	2 slices

1. Combine the ingredients, mixing them together well.
2. Spread the filling onto the bread.

Egg and Celery
CHO 30g/kcalories 130

1	egg, hard-boiled	1
1 stick	celery, finely chopped	1 stick
1 x 15ml sp/ 1 tbs	reduced-calorie mayonnaise	1 tbs
2 slices	wholemeal bread	2 slices

1. Mix the ingredients together, combining them well.
2. Spread the filling onto the bread.

Tuna and Mayonnaise
CHO 30g/kcalories 200

100g/4oz	tinned tuna in brine, drained	⅔ cup
2 x 15ml sp/ 2 tbs	reduced-calorie mayonnaise	2 tbs
	salt and freshly ground black pepper	
	a few slices cucumber and/or tomato	
2 slices	wholemeal bread	2 slices

1. Combine the ingredients, mixing them well.
2. Spread the filling onto the bread.

WELSH RAREBIT

CHO 60g/kcalories 580
Serves 4

Metric/Imperial		*American*
4 slices	wholemeal bread	4 slices
100g/4oz	reduced-fat cheddar cheese, grated	1 cup
pinch	paprika	pinch
1 x 5ml sp/1 tsp	mustard powder	1 tsp
1 x 5ml sp/1 tsp	Worcestershire sauce	1 tsp

1. Toast the bread on one side under the grill.
2. Meanwhile, combine the remaining ingredients. Spread the cheese mixture on the untoasted side of the bread and grill gently for 3–4 minutes until the cheese is bubbling and golden brown. Serve immediately.

AMERICAN-STYLE HAMBURGERS

CHO 100g/kcalories 1270
Serves 4

Metric/Imperial		*American*
450g/1 lb	extra lean mince beef	1lb
50g/2oz	wholemeal breadcrumbs	1 cup
1 x 5ml sp/1 tsp	mixed herbs	1 tsp
	salt and freshly ground	
	black pepper	
1	size 3 egg, beaten	1
4	hamburger buns	4
4	lettuce leaves	4
2	tomatoes, sliced	2
1	onion, sliced	1

1. Put the minced beef, breadcrumbs and herbs into a bowl and mix them together well. Season to taste with salt and freshly ground black pepper, then bind the mixture together with the egg. Shape the mixture into 4 thick burgers and chill until needed.
2. Grill the burgers under medium heat for about 8 minutes on each side, or until they have cooked all the way through but aren't too dry. Then, split the buns and put a lettuce leaf and tomato and onion slices on the bottom half of each, put a burger on top then replace the other half of the bun.

HAM AND MUSHROOM STUFFED
BAKED POTATOES

CHO 00g/kcalories 000
Serves 4

Metric/Imperial		*American*
4 medium	potatoes, cleaned	4 medium
25g/1oz	low-fat spread	2 tbs
1	onion, peeled and chopped	1
100g/4oz	mushrooms, chopped	1½ cups
	salt and freshly ground black pepper	
50g/2oz	lean ham, chopped	2 tbs
50g/2oz	reduced-fat cheddar cheese, grated	½ cup

1. Bake the potatoes at 400°F/200°C/gas mark 6 for 45 minutes to 1 hour, or until the potatoes are soft all the way through.
2. Towards the end of the potatoes' cooking time, melt the low-fat spread in a pan and sauté the onion and mushrooms. Season to taste and stir in the ham and grated cheese.
3. Cut the potatoes in half lengthways and scoop out the cooked flesh into a bowl, making sure that you do not pierce the skins. Mash it well, beat in the mushroom mixture, then spoon it back into the potato skins and return them to the oven and bake for a further 10–15 minutes.

Ideas for Children

PIZZA

CHO 150g/kcalories 1090
Serves 4–6

Metric/Imperial		*American*
Base		
225g/8oz	wholemeal self-raising flour	2 cups
1 x 5ml sp/1 tsp	baking powder	1 tsp
pinch	salt	pinch
25g/1oz	low-fat spread	2 tbs
25g/1oz	reduced-fat cheddar, grated	¼ cup
150ml/¼ pint	skimmed milk	⅔ cup
Topping		
2 x 15ml sp/ 2 tbs	tomato purée	2 tbs
1	onion, peeled and finely chopped	1
pinch	dried mixed herbs	pinch
50g/2oz	button mushrooms, sliced	¾ cup
50g/2oz	reduced-fat cheddar, grated	½ cup

1. Sieve the flour and baking powder into a bowl. Add the pinch of salt and the low-fat spread and rub them in until the mixture resembles coarse breadcrumbs.

Stir in the cheese, then add the milk and mix until you have a rough dough.

2. Turn it out onto a floured surface and knead it until the dough is smooth. Roll it out on a lightly floured surface to form a 23cm/9 inch round, then transfer it to a lightly greased baking sheet.

3. Now add the topping. Spread the tomato purée over the surface, sprinkle on the onion and herbs, add the mushrooms, then sprinkle the cheese over the top.

4. Bake the pizza at 425°F/220°C/gas mark 7 for 20–25 minutes or until the cheese is bubbling and golden brown.

STRAWBERRY AND YOGURT JELLY

CHO 10g/kcalories 90
Serves 4–6

Metric/Imperial		American
1	packet strawberry-flavour sugar-free jelly crystals	1
1 x 150g/5fl oz	carton diet strawberry yogurt	⅔ cup

1. Make up the jelly according to the directions on the packet and leave it to cool until it just starts to start, then fold in the yogurt. Pour the mixture into a wetted 550ml/1 pint mould or bowl, then chill in the refrigerator until it has set firm.
2. You can turn the jelly out onto a serving dish if you want to – just dip the mould in very hot water for a couple of seconds, invert the serving dish and put it on top of the mould, then, holding the plate tightly over it, turn it quickly and then lift the mould off.

JELLY CASTLES

CHO 30g/kcalories 370
Serves 4

Metric/Imperial		*American*
1	packet orange-flavour sugar-free jelly crystals	1
4 x 15ml sp/ 4 tbs	desiccated coconut	4 tbs
1 x 300g/10½oz	can mandarin oranges in natural juice	1¼ cups

1. Rinse out 4 150ml/¼ pint moulds or empty yogurt cartons with cold water.
2. Make up the jelly according to the directions on the packet and pour equal amounts of the mixture into the wetted moulds. Cover them with clingfilm and chill until the jellies have set.
3. Unmould the jellies into individual dishes, dipping them briefly into very hot water.
4. Sprinkle the tops and sides of the jellies with the coconut and arrange all but 4 of the mandarin segments around the bottom edge of the jellies. Decorate the top of each jelly with a mandarin segment.
5. Chill the Jelly Castles until you are ready to serve.

Note to Cooks

Use whichever flavour your child likes best and decorate with the appropriate fruit.

PEAR MICE

CHO 40g/kcalories 180
Makes 6–7

Metric/Imperial		American
1	packet sugar-free jelly crystals	1
1 x 400g/14oz	tin pear halves in natural juice, drained and the juice reserved	1¾ cups
18–21	currants	18–21
	strip angelica	

1. Make the jelly as per the instructions on the packet, using the pear juice made up to the amount given with water. Chill the jelly in the refrigerator until it has set.
2. Roughly chop the jelly and arrange it on a plate. Put the pear halves on the jelly, cut side down – these are the mice! Press the currants into the fruit so that each 'mouse' has 2 'eyes' and a 'nose'. Cut the angelica into very fine strips and stick a few into each side of the nose to make whiskers.

Note to Cooks

This is ideal for children's parties and very easy to make.

CARIBBEAN DRINK

CHO 50g/kcalories 220
Serves 4

Metric/Imperial		*American*
1	canned pineapple ring, in natural juice, drained	1
2 small	bananas, peeled	2 small
1 wineglass	unsweetened orange juice	1 wineglass
1	lime, juice of	1
approx. 150ml/¼ pint	diet pineapple and grapefruit drink	⅔ cup
	about 6 ice cubes	

1. Put all the ingredients into a blender or liquidizer and process until the mixture is smooth.
2. Pour into 4 glasses and serve immediately.

PEACH AND GINGER FIZZ

CHO 30g/kcalories 130
Serves 4

Metric/Imperial		*American*
2 medium	peaches, peeled, stoned and chopped	2 medium
1 wineglass	unsweetened apple juice	1 wineglass
1 x 550ml/ 1 pint	bottle slimline ginger ale	2½ cups
	crushed ice	

1. Put the peaches and apple juice in a blender or liquid-izer and process until the mixture is smooth. Add the ginger ale.
2. Put the crushed ice into 4 glasses and pour out the drink. Serve immediately.

STRAWBERRY MILKSHAKE

CHO 10g/kcalories 120
Serves 2

Metric/Imperial		*American*
275ml/½ pint	skimmed milk	1⅓ cups
100g/4oz	strawberries, hulled if fresh, thawed if frozen	1 cup
1 x 5ml sp/1 tsp	intense artificial sweetener (optional)	1 tsp

1. Put the milk, strawberries and sweetener in a blender or liquidizer and process for 15–20 seconds.
2. Strain the Milkshake into 2 glasses and serve immediately.

Useful Addresses

United Kingdom
British Diabetic Association, 10 Queen Anne Street,
London W1M 0BD
0171 323 1531

USA
American Diabetes Association, 1660 Duke Street,
Alexandria, VA 22314
1-703 549 1500
1-800 232 3472 (USA Only)

Australia
Diabeties Australia, QBE Building, 33–35 Ainslie
Avenue, Canberra ACT, PO Box 944, Civic Square ACT
2608
61 62 475655
61 62 475722

Austria
Österreichischer Diabetikervereinigung, (Austrian Diabetes Association), Moosstrasse 18, 5020 Salzburg
43 222 82 09 753

Belgium
Belgische Vereniging voor Suikerzieken, (Belgian Association for Diabetics), BVS Secretariat, Charles de Kerchovelaan 369, B-9000 Ghent
32 91 20 05 20

Canada
Canadian Diabetes Association, 78 Bond Street, Toronto, Ontario M5B 2J8
1-416 362 4440

Czechoslovakia
Czechoslovak Diabetology Association, Internal Clinic ILF, National Diabetes Program, Coordinating Centre, 762 75 Gottwaldov
42 28235

Denmark
Diabetesforeningen (Danish Diabetes Association), Filosofgangen 24, 5000 Odense C
45 66 129006

Finland
Suomen Diabetesliitto r.y. Diabetesförbundet i Finland r.f. (Finnish Diabetes Association), Diabeteskeskus,

Kirjoniementie 15, SF-33680 Tampere
358 31 600 333

France
Association Française des Diabétiques, 14 rue du Clos,
75020 Paris
331-40 08 24 25

Germany
Deutscher Diabetiker-Bund e.V. (German Diabetes
Union), Danzigerweg 1, D-5880 Lüdenscheid
49 2351 85053

Greece
Panhellenic Diabetic Association, Feidiou Street 18,
Athens
30 1 362 9717

Hungary
Magyar Diabetes Társagág (Hungarian Diabetes
Association), Korányi S. utca 2a, Budapest 1083
36 1 330 360

Ireland
Irish Diabetic Association, 82/83 Lower Gardiner Street,
Dublin 1
363022

Italy
Associazione Italiana per la Difesa Degli, Interesi di
Diabetici, Via del Scrofa 14, Roma
39 2 654 3784

Grand-Duché de Luxembourg
Association Luxembourgeoise du Diabète, PO Box
1316, Luxembourg
352 474545
352 4411 1

Netherlands
Diabetes Vereniging Nederland (Dutch Diabetes
Association), Puntenburgerlaan 91, 3812 CC, Amersfoort
31 33 63 05 66

Norway
Norges Diabetesforbund (Norwegian Diabetes
Association), Østensjøveien 29, 0661 Oslo 6
47 2 65 45 50

Poland
Polskie Towarzystwo Diabetologiczne (Polish Diabet-
ological Association), Kopernika 17, 31-501 Kraków
48 12 21 01 44
48 12 21 40 54

Portugal
Associaçao Protectora dos Diabéticos de Portugal (Portuguese Diabetic Association), Rua do Salitre, 118, 1200 Lisbon
351 1 680041 (42)
351 2 682729

Spain
Sociedad Espanola de Diabetes (Spanish Diabetes Society), Colegio Official de Médicos, Santa Isabel, 51, 28012 Madrid
341 2396519

Sweden
Svenska Endokrinolog föreningen (Swedish Society of Endocrinology), Department of Internal Medicine, University Hospital, S-75185 Uppsala
46 18 663000

Switzerland
(Switzerische Diabetes) Gesellschaft (Swiss Diabetes Association), Hegarstrasse 18, CH-8032 Zurich
41 1 383 13 15

Yugoslavia
Savez Drustava za Zastitu od Secerne Bolesti (The Association of Diabetic Societies of Yugoslavia), 4a Dugi Dol, PO Box 958, 41000 Zagreb
38 41 232 222
38 41 231 480

Further Reading

Day, Dr John, *The Diabetes Handbook, Insulin dependent diabetes* (1st Edition), Thorsons, 1986

Day, Dr John, *The Diabetes Handbook, Non-insulin dependent diabetes* (2nd Edition), British Diabetic Association, 1992

Govindji, Azmina and Jill Myers, *Diabetic Entertaining*, Thorsons, 1990

North, Judith, *Teenage Diabetes*, Thorsons, 1990

Sönksen, Peter, Charles Fox and Sue Judd, *Diabetes at your fingertips* (3rd Edition), Class Publishing, 1994

British Diabetic Association

DIABETES AFFECTS just over two per cent of the UK population. Although it cannot be cured or prevented, it can be controlled by proper treatment. There may be times when you need advice or information and this is where the BDA can help.

The BDA is an independent registered charity with over 140,000 members and 400 local branches. It represents people with diabetes, liaising with Government Departments and professional bodies on matters concerning diabetes.

The Association provides information and practical advice for people with diabetes and their families. A wide range of literature, goods and videos are available on all aspects of diabetes.

The BDA's magazine, *Balance*, is published every two months and is sent free to members or is available from newsagents. It keeps readers up to date with the latest medical news, local events and include articles on living with diabetes. All people with diabetes are advised to eat healthily and *Balance* gives recipes and dietary information to help bring interest and variety to diabetic eating.

The Association also supports research to improve treatments and to find a prevention or cure for diabetes. Currently spending around £3.5 million each year, the BDA is the largest single contributor dedicated to diabetic research.

For over 60 years, the BDA has strived to achieve its aims, but it has only been able to do so with the help of its members and supporters. Please join the BDA. For further details and an application form, contact:

British Diabetic Association
10 Queen Anne Street
London W1M 0BD
United Kingdom
Tel: 0171–323 1531

Index